MACULAR
DISEASE

MACULAR DISEASE

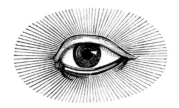

Practical Strategies for Living with Vision Loss

2nd Edition

Peggy R. Wolfe

PARK PUBLISHING, INC.
Minneapolis, Minnesota
New Richmond, Wisconsin

Second edition

Printed in the United States of America

ISBN: 978-0-9792945-2-5

Library of Congress Cataloging-in-Publication data
Wolfe, Peggy R.
    Macular disease : practical strategies for living with vision loss / Peggy R. Wolfe. — 2nd ed.
        p. cm.
    Includes index.
    ISBN 978-0-9792945-2-5 (pbk.)
    1. Retinal degeneration—Popular works.   2. Low vision—Handbooks, manuals, etc.   I. Title.
    RE661.D3W65 2011
    617.7'35—dc23

                                                            2011026839

Editor: Marly Cornell
Cover and interior designer: Monica Baziuk
Photography: Scott Knutson and Steven F. Wolfe
Indexer: Robert J. Richardson

Product photographs and trademarks are used in this book for informational purposes only. This book is not endorsed or sponsored by, or otherwise affiliated with, any of the manufacturers or trademark owners.

PARK PUBLISHING, INC.
511 Wisconsin Drive
New Richmond, Wisconsin 54017

9 8 7 6 5 4 3 2 1

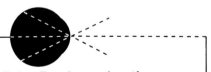

This Large Print Book carries the
Seal of Approval of N.A.V.H.

Contents

---

4. Nurturing Your Body   41

PART 2
Using Practical Hints
to Make Your Life Easier   61

5. Cooking and Eating Use
Senses of Touch and Hearing   63

PART 3
Arranging Your Affairs and Using Assistive Technology 119

8. Dealing with Financial, Personal, and Legal Affairs 121

9. Embracing Technology 141

About this book's design

THIS TRULY large print book was designed specifically for the reader who has limited vision. My goal was to find a typeface that would be easy to read and a layout that would clearly identify the topics. The first step was research on the readability of serif vs. sans serif typefaces. Serifs are small decorative lines added as embellishment to the ends of strokes in letters. Research revealed that the less fancy, more open letters and numerals in sans serif fonts are easier for people with low vision to read than serif fonts. Consider the difficulty you may have had in knowing whether a numeral is a 6 or a 9. In the open font of this book, it is easier to distinguish the two numbers than it is in many serif fonts.

The next decision was choosing the easiest to read sans serif font. After testing several fonts with low vision readers who were members of support groups, this Frutiger font was named the winner. Designed by Adrian

Frutiger for signage in the Charles de Gaulle airport in Paris, where the installation was completed in 1975, the font is known for its legibility. For this reason, Frutiger has been used in many other ways in addition to airport signs.

Low vision readers expressed preference for the large type size used in the book and in the layout features, including the headings that indicate new topics. Readers were quite firm about placing the page numbers at the bottom of the page, in the center.

The book is printed on glare-resistant, heavy paper that makes the pages durable and easy to turn. The off-white color provides good contrast against the large, heavy, black type.

The designer and the author hope that you enjoy handling and reading this book.

Preface to the 2nd edition

IN THE THREE YEARS since the publication of the first edition, I've learned many new things from people I've met and from personal trial and error. There has been great progress in the treatment of wet macular degeneration, improving the outlook for people with this condition. My goal is to provide hope along with useful hints to others on my same path.

This revision is again being written in real time as I continue to adjust to the progressive decline of my vision from macular degeneration. I was diagnosed in 1999, at the relatively "young" age of sixty-nine.

I was referred by my ophthalmologist to a retinologist, and the diagnosis of early macular degeneration was confirmed. I wasn't too surprised, as my mother and my uncle lived with macular disease for many years. They provided me with gutsy examples of how to live with vision loss. Longtime exposure to their stalwart optimism left me with an accepting spirit—one filled not with fear, but with the will to do battle. I've fought vision loss by developing strategies to make my life easier now, and to prepare for the day when I may have to rely solely on my peripheral vision.

In 2005, I asked my retinologist how much longer he predicted I'd be able to read. Taken aback by my question, he blurted out "one to two years." Rather than discouraging me, this news energized me to accelerate my preparation and to share what I've learned with others in the same situation. I hope you will find the ideas presented in this book useful. Because macular diseases generally proceed slowly, I hope this book can be your handy companion for many years.

Peggy R. Wolfe

Introduction

MY GOAL with this book is to offer hope, confidence, and optimism to those with progressive vision loss. Aimed particularly at people with one of the many macular diseases—the most common are macular degeneration and diabetic retinopathy—this book offers useful tips and strategies for anyone with vision loss. Family and friends can also gain insight and understanding of the challenges faced by their loved ones. A "You can do it" approach offers a positive way of looking at life now and later as we continue to learn about attitudes and aids that can help us along the way.

As a lay person whose expertise comes from having lived with vision loss from macular degeneration since 1999, I do not attempt to address the medical aspects of macular disease. Rather, the book is a personal guide to dealing with the real situations and challenges that you have now or may encounter in the future. You will find that, although you may need to do things differently, you can still do them. Those of us with vision loss experience both trials and triumphs, and many of mine are illustrated here in the form of personal stories about experiences I have had as I learned, and continue to learn, to live with macular degeneration.

For a quick overview of the topics covered in the book, look through the table of contents, or skim through the chapters to get an idea of what is covered. Then read those sections that seem most relevant to your life right now. Or you may prefer to read the book from cover to cover and follow the story of my life with diminishing vision. I suggest you keep this book in an easy-to-find spot so that you can refer to it whenever a new situation comes up. As you face a new challenge, look in the index for topics that will help you deal with the new problem. Use these ideas as the starting points to develop your own techniques for a better life.

PART 1

Sustaining the Spirit, Mind, and Body

"YOU CAN DO IT" is the message of this book. Using your mind and your spirit, you can discover ways to enjoy your life now and prepare for the future. Chapter 1 offers a positive approach to living with vision loss. Chapters 2, 3, and 4 describe ways to maximize your vision with special lighting, care for your body through diet and exercise, optimize hearing (despite some loss), and develop your sense of touch and other senses.

Personal **"MY STORY"** features are inserted throughout the book to illustrate both the author's triumphs and mishaps.

Nourishing the Spirit and the Mind

YOUR LIFE, after receiving a diagnosis of a macular disease, will likely take a different course from the one you had expected, but it is not a hopeless picture. You will find you can still do the things you have been doing—but you will need to do them in different ways. You have the power to be active in finding solutions to the particular difficulties you may face. Do not think of yourself as a victim of the disease. Instead, recognize yourself as a fighter who will use creative problem solving to meet the challenges posed by vision loss. Make finding tactics to deal with the realities of the disease your strategic game plan. You can use ideas in this book that have worked for others to find solutions that work for you.

Strengthen your spirit

What do we mean by "spirit"? People think of spirit in many different ways. One definition is "life force." Helpful qualities within that concept include: backbone, boldness, character, dauntlessness, energy, enterprise, enthusiasm, grit, guts, heart, humor, morale, motivation, resolve, soul, vitality, warmth, and will. Developing these inner resources will help you live a rewarding life with courage and purpose.

Develop positive attitudes and deal with stress

Consider the following qualities as gifts that will help you develop the strong spirit that will lead to a positive outlook: acceptance and patience, powerfulness, enthusiasm and enjoyment, and most important, gratitude. Think of how you can use these qualities to enhance your day.

Acceptance and patience

Realize that life involves change and yours will include limitations that you didn't expect. As certain everyday things take longer than before, you will be able to meet new challenges more effectively if you can nurture a sense of calm. You may need to allow yourself to grieve your losses while moving on to acceptance. Understand that you are dealing not only with the loss of vision, but also the loss of what you thought the rest of your life would be like. As with any other grief, you may feel shock or disbelief, or even find yourself in denial that this is happening to you. Anger, fear, and questions of "Why me?" are other common reactions.

You may experience a profound sadness and have trouble dealing with anxiety about the future. These are normal and understandable emotions, and allowing yourself to feel them can help you to accept what is happening and then to let go of your fears. If your vision loss—which perhaps comes on top of other losses—causes you significant depression, it may help you, as it has helped others, to seek counseling or a vision loss support group. Be patient and gentle with yourself as you strive for acceptance every new day—it will bring you both peace and the will to move forward to your new "normal" life.

Powerfulness

Many things in life have always been beyond our control, from the forces of nature to the behavior of others. Being confronted with some new limitations in life does not mean you are suddenly less powerful. Know that you still have control over how you live your life. There are still many parts of life that you can control. The most important thing is your attitude. If you are discouraged, counter that feeling with a determination to rule your own life. As diseases affecting the macula usually have a slow progression, you may well have years of quite functional, albeit declining, vision. Consider your diagnosis an advance notice—a gift of time to gradually prepare for the day that could come when you may have to rely only on your peripheral vision. Use this book as a guide to highlighting things you can do in various areas of your life to maintain the independence that will bolster your confidence and sense of power.

Enthusiasm and enjoyment

Be good to yourself and do what is most important to you. At first, most people who receive a diagnosis of macular disease feel confused, frightened, and depressed. I suggest that the first thing to do in that uncertain time is to figure out what are the most important things in your life—the things that bring you the most contentment and joy. Then immediately plan to do one of these things as a special treat to yourself. Choose something that fills your heart with joy. Practical activities required for daily living don't qualify. What you pick need not involve a financial expenditure, but rather the investment and the reward of love and time well spent. Take a walk with a friend in a beautiful park or visit someone you haven't seen in a long time. Enjoy a museum or go to a concert with a friend.

You can save most of your ideas for later times, but this first one should be something really special. Then remember to find ways to be good to yourself on a continuing basis. Find ways to relax and enjoy what you are doing. Have some special fun and develop your mind. If you want to meet people and learn new things, seek out activities at senior centers—get on their mailing list for their newsletters with monthly calendars of events. Take an adult enrichment class offered by your school district that can exercise your mind as well as your body. Local low vision agencies offer many fun classes and excursions. Maybe your idea of fun and relaxation is simply a slower pace to your life so that you can savor each day. If you haven't already, now is the time to develop computer skills. You can keep in touch with grandchildren via email, find the latest news on the Internet, and find information on any subject, play games—and much more.

Gratitude

Perhaps the most important of all is gratitude. Think of the things in your life for which you are thankful. I am thankful for—

- the gift of time to find ways to remain as independent as possible.

- willingness to ask for help when needed (still hard for me).

- family and friends who graciously help with tasks and transportation.

- stabilization of the vision in my right "good" eye following injections.

- continuing research into developing new ways to treat macular degeneration.

Stress reduction

A common reaction to vision loss—which can include events such as taking twice as long to perform a task as before or beginning to acknowledge that you should stop driving—is stress. The body frequently expresses stress in the forms of headache, stomachache, or trouble sleeping. There are times when you feel particularly harried or frustrated or sad and may want to bury those feelings. Instead, here are some methods to deal with your stress:

- Talk about it with those around you. If you are alone, call a family member or friend. The important thing is to talk about it.

- Realize that stress is contagious—if you are feeling stressed, chances are good that those around you will begin to feel stressed. If you are all trying to ignore, deny, or bottle up your feelings, you end up with a group of inwardly seething, frustrated people.

- Tell people if you are overwhelmed and need help, rather than wondering why they can't see that you need help.

- Recognize that a grief expressed is a grief diminished.

- Take a break.

- Know that it's OK to yell or cry.

- Help someone else.

The best way to prevent stress from building up is, of course, to prevent it from taking hold in the first place. Here are some ways to ward off stress in your life.

- Be patient and accepting of yourself.

- Know your limits and set realistic goals when you plan your day.

- Take frequent breaks by stretching and deep breathing.

- Refuse to hold grudges or feel sorry for yourself.

- Get enough sleep.

- Exercise regularly.

- Meditate or regularly engage in the practices of your belief system.

- Laugh often, even if you don't feel like doing so. Smiling relaxes the muscles in your face.

——————— MY STORY ———————

Dream Trip with My Daughter
After a Scary Prognosis

When my retinologist told me he guessed I had one to two years before I lost my central vision, meaning I'd no longer be able to read, I sat down and thought about how this new situation would fit into my life. I decided the first step was to figure out what was most important to me. The answer was twofold—first, to spend time with my daughter, who lives in another state; and second, to experience the great joys of my life—classical music, opera, ballet, and visual arts. This all added up to a trip with my daughter to New York City. It was a special time together, and we visited art museums and attended opera and ballet performances. We shared all expenses, which helped to make the trip possible, and I will always have the memory of our time together doing things we both love.

Nurture your mind

Keep your mind active by reading if you are able. You can get books and magazines in large print versions as reading becomes more difficult. If you listen to the radio or TV with your eyes closed, you can develop your listening skills. Get used to listening to books on tape or compact discs or as downloads from the Internet—this skill will come in handy, as you can become eligible to participate in the free Talking Book Program, a service of the Library of Congress, which is described on pages 142–146.

Learn something new by taking classes offered by community education organizations and low vision agencies. Most offer courses on how to use a computer, how to access the Internet and use email. For one-on-one instruction, ask your children, grandchildren, or friends to teach you. Developing computer skills will open untold doors for you, and technological advances in accessibility are making computers easier and easier to use.

Find a spiritual home

For many people, belonging to a faith community brings spiritual fulfillment and peace. Membership in churches, synagogues, or other places of worship can lead you to fellowship with people who give you comfort and support. Study groups and classes are often offered. If you have not already found such a spiritual home but feel a yearning, this is a good time to start that search.

Volunteer for rich rewards

Perhaps the best thing you can do for yourself, while helping others at the same time, is to become a volunteer. You may think you have nothing to offer, but there is an opportunity waiting for you somewhere. Churches, the United Way, and senior centers are three good places to find the right volunteer work for you. These organizations need volunteers for all types of jobs, so think about your skills and what you enjoy doing, and make a call. If there is a vision rehabilitation center in your community, you can join an advocacy group or work with a staff member in a support group. The possibilities are endless.

———————————— MY STORY ————————————

First a New Church, Then a Perfect Volunteer Job

I had halfheartedly been looking for a spiritual home over a period of years. I'd attend one church for a few months, then another. I did not feel at home in any of them. Then one Sunday I attended services at a church that I'd been hearing had beautiful music. I had not gone there before because I thought it was too huge a congregation, but as soon as I felt the friendly atmosphere and heard the soloist and choir, I knew this was where I belonged. My search was over and I joined the church right away. Soon I wanted to be more closely involved in its community, so I started looking for a volunteer job among the many offerings.

One day the coordinator called, said there was an opening in the music library, and asked if I'd be interested, considering I had a library degree. I said yes, and was soon working with a special woman who has become my "volunteer buddy." Our project is to list in a database each track of the hundreds of compact discs held by members of the music department. Our trio of coordinator and two volunteer buddies has developed a close and loving relationship that is important to each of us. My friendship with these two women has enriched my life beyond words, and the bonus is that I'm working with music, too. These have been great gifts to me.

Caring for Your Eyes and Vision

MONITOR YOUR VISION regularly and if you notice changes, see your doctor right away. Take good care of your eyes to keep seeing at the highest possible level.

Do home vision tests if you have macular degeneration

Annual checkups are not enough if you have macular degeneration, because you are responsible for monitoring your sight on a regular basis. You can do simple tests at home. Your eye doctor may have directed you to use an Amsler grid to check your own eyes periodically. Make the grid test a habit by doing it in the same location, with the same lighting, and at about the same time of day, so you can more accurately compare your results with those of previous tests. Be aware of what you see with each eye in order to notice any changes since your previous test.

There are other important ways to monitor your sight. Develop your own benchmark system to check your vision in each eye. For example, you can test your vision by looking, with each eye, at a bedside clock, your watch, or the bathroom scale, or by reading with each eye to see if the lines are wavy. Choose something that you read every day or at least every week, such as a TV guide, a newspaper, or a program for religious services. Also, take note if you suddenly need more light for a particular task or if you develop a new sensitivity to glare. Take a proactive approach to monitoring your vision, and take fast action if you notice a change that could require immediate treatment.

Contact your doctor if you notice a change in your vision

Although at the time of this writing in 2011 there is no treatment for the dry type of macular degeneration, there are treatments for the wet type, and promising research is being conducted on treatments for both types. Treatments are also available for other diseases that affect the macula.

If you notice a change in either eye:

- Act immediately, in time for helpful treatment.
- If you have trouble getting an immediate appointment, be an advocate for yourself and keep insisting that you see the doctor.
- Do not procrastinate!

Visit your eye doctors regularly for checkups and tests

When dealing with macular disease, it is important to have complete eye examinations every year with a retinologist who specializes in retinal and macular diseases. You may be directed to have more frequent appointments. See an ophthalmologist on an annual basis for a general eye checkup and for a possible adjustment to the prescription for your eyeglasses.

Carry a copy of your eyeglass prescriptions, along with the phone numbers of both your ophthalmologist and retinologist, in case you lose or break your glasses when you are out of town. If you have a sudden change in vision when you are away, be prepared to call your retinologist for advice and a possible referral to a doctor in the vicinity. For a longer stay away from home, be prepared with the name and contact information of a retinologist that your doctor recommends. The new doctor can call your regular retinologist to obtain your history, including treatments you have received.

At retinology appointments your distance vision is checked by reading rows of letters on a distant chart. Near vision may be checked by reading from a small card you hold in your hand that has rows of text or numbers in decreasing sizes of type. This card tests the vision for reading and other close work. If you have macular degeneration, you may be asked to check your eyes with an Amsler grid, like you use at home. These vision tests are usually followed by a glaucoma test. You are given drops to dilate your pupils so the doctor can see into the back of your eyes.

Depending on your diagnosis, further tests may be conducted. At an initial visit, two types of photographs may be taken with a special camera. One type takes color photos. The other is fluorescein angiography, which involves injecting a dye into a vein in your hand or arm. As the dye circulates through the bloodstream and eventually reaches the eye, the blood vessels in the retina become visible to the special camera, which takes flash photographs of the eye every few seconds for several minutes. These photo sessions can be uncomfortable due to the bright light that is flashed into your eyes, but the photos help the doctor determine changes or abnormal blood vessels. The fine detail shown in the photos, when enlarged, makes the fluorescein angiography an accurate and valuable tool for the diagnosis of many eye conditions.

Another test, called ocular coherence tomography (OCT) but informally called a scan, obtains high-resolution cross-sectional images of the retina. This is used in the diagnosis of a host of macular diseases and to follow up on responses to various types of treatment. For example, if you have macular degeneration and bleeding is suspected, or if you have had injections in your eye, you will probably have OCT scans at each visit. The scans take just moments and there is no discomfort as there are no bright flashes of light.

Shortly after the tests, the doctor visually examines your eyes, and checks and explains your test results. Having someone present with you is an advantage so that you do not miss something important. Come prepared with a written list of questions and take notes of the doctor's responses to your questions for later review. It is easy to forget when there is a lot of information. Ask your companion to write down information the doctor gives about results of your tests, possible treatments, and suggestions for home care. At my own visits, a number of different people have come as my support person—my husband, son, daughter, and a cousin from Ireland who was in the country and who also had an appointment. These visits also help your family members understand your disease and how it is progressing.

——————— MY STORY ———————

Bleeding in the Right Eye—
and Then the Left?

I used to think that the telltale sign of bleeding in the eye would be some wild vision distortion such as seeing a clock face as twisted, or print in a book or newspaper as a blur of crooked lines. But my retinologist always ended each visit by asking that I call if I noticed even a small change in either eye.

On my 77th birthday I was feeling confident because I'd passed the vision test for renewing my driver's license two weeks earlier, much to my surprise. Yet I was trying not to admit to myself that something had changed in my right, "good," eye. That Sunday at church, where I gratefully use the large print program, for the first time I found that I could not read the ends of lines or see the music to sing. At home, glare from my computer screen had become intense. I had to change to different types of lightbulbs in the dining room, where I have my morning coffee while I read the newspaper—which had suddenly become quite blurry with wavy lines. I was able to pinpoint the problem to my right eye because I was in the habit of testing my vision by reading the daily paper first with one eye, then the other. I usually did vision checks throughout each day, too, by looking at stationary distant objects.

I was afraid to make the call to the doctor, but my son's words about the importance of caring for my vision kept ringing in my ears. I made the call after a few days.

My retinologist looked at my dilated right eye and said he saw bleeding, the sign that I now had wet macular degeneration. To confirm the diagnosis, he ordered a fluorescein angiogram and an OTC scan. The diagnosis was confirmed. The doctor said he was surprised, because I was young to have developed the wet form of macular degeneration. He said he was amazed that I'd noticed the change because the bleeding was so slight, and he bemoaned the people who don't notice changes or put off seeing a doctor for six months—at which point, treatment is less able to help.

Before I left the office, treatment was started. I received an injection of Avastin in my right eye that we hoped would halt the bleeding so that my sight would stay at its present level. Almost immediately my vision actually improved, and when I went for my six-week checkup and another injection, we found that my vision had improved to the point that it had been before the bleeding. At the twelve-week point, my vision had continued to improve, but I had another injection as planned. At the six-month point, my right eye vision remained stable. I had no further bleeding until three years later, in 2010, when I then had a series of Avastin injections. Each month, the OTC scan showed improvement and finally I was able to discontinue the injections.

My left eye has not developed bleeding, but degeneration of the cells in the macula has accelerated to a point where I am legally blind in my left eye.

Special vitamins for macular degeneration

The National Eye Institute's "Age-Related Eye Disease Study" resulted in a vitamin supplement known as the AREDS formula. There are different varieties of the AREDS formula. The original formula contained beta-carotene (vitamin A), but not lutein (another naturally occurring carotenoid that aids in eyesight). A newer formula contained lutein, but not beta-carotene. Ask your doctor which formula is right for you.

—————————— **MY STORY** ——————————

Sisters in Separate
Five-year Research Studies

When I was diagnosed at my first visit in 1999, the retinologist told me about a research study that was testing low-level laser surgery as a way to slow the progress of macular degeneration. When he asked if I'd like to join the study, I immediately agreed. I've always been interested in research; and I knew that, even if it didn't help me, it could help others. I was the third patient in the practice to sign on. After I qualified for the study, the doctor received a sealed envelope that held a piece of paper with my name and either "Right eye" or "Left eye." I was hoping it would be my left eye that had been randomly selected because the right eye had better vision, but the patient had no choice. Following the laser treatment, my eyes were checked every six months for five years by a research coordinator who did special tests.

The results of multiple studies of low-level laser treatment showed no statistical advantage over not receiving any treatment.

As it happened, my sister was a participant at the same time in a completely different study that tested the particular vitamin-antioxidant combination in the AREDS formula. It was this study that showed positive results. Taking the special formula slowed the progress of macular disease in some cases. Doctors then started to recommend taking AREDS pills on a daily basis.

Protect your eyes from the sun

It is generally recommended that you protect your eyes from the sun. If you are affected by glare, such protection is necessary for your comfort. Glare is also a problem for some people when they are in a car and even when they are indoors. Wide-brimmed and visor hats and sunglasses can provide protection. The best type of sunglasses is also among the least expensive.

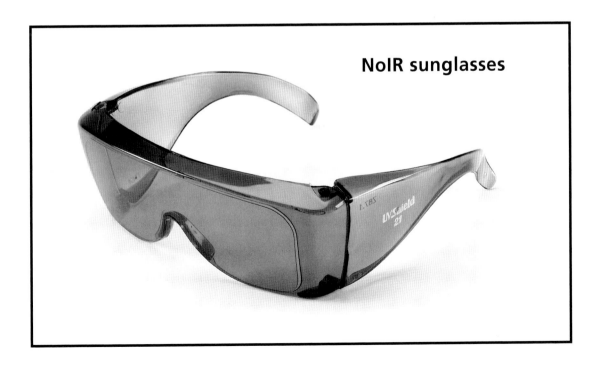

NoIR sunglasses

These NoIR sunglasses come in both fit-over and wraparound styles. They offer 100 percent ultraviolet protection. They also help prevent glare and block blue light. The wraparound model shown here is excellent because it prevents sunlight from coming in from the sides. The sunglasses are reasonably priced and come in various sizes and lens colors. The color to select depends on your eye condition, as different colors are recommended for diabetic retinopathy, macular degeneration, and retinitis pigmentosa. Visit the NoIR website to see photos of the various colors available. A large selection of NoIR sunglasses is available through the low vision stores listed in Appendix A, and some of these stores' catalogs have helpful charts showing suitable sunglasses colors for various eye diseases. These low vision stores carry many other useful products, and you'll find many references to them throughout the book. I suggest you order a catalog right now.

Get both reading and distance glasses

Having the proper glasses for both near-sight activities (such as reading, writing checks, and sewing) and far-sight activities (such as driving and watching television), allows you to have maximum field of vision at both far and close distances. If you currently wear bifocal or trifocal glasses, you may benefit from separate reading and distance glasses. I also have "computer" glasses that are set for the distance between my eyes and the computer monitor.

Keep your glasses clean

A smudge on your glasses can cause a big scare. Often when I start to read it seems that my vision has suddenly gone. But when I hold my glasses up to the light, I see smudges and specks. I wear my reading glasses on a chain around my neck, and the way the lenses hang down seems to make them a magnet for specks and dust. I clean the lenses frequently and place bottles of glasses cleaner in every room so it is easy to clean my glasses. Get tall bottles so you'll be able to spot them standing upright.

Fix drooping eyebrows and eyelids with surgery covered by Medicare

As we age, upper eyelids sometimes droop and block the upper field of vision. This can give the appearance of half-open eyes. One cause of drooping is reduced tone in the muscles that control the eyelids. This condition can also be caused by eyebrows that droop so much that they make the eyelids droop as well. If this drooping limits your field of vision, Medicare may cover approved surgical procedures to correct the problem. A direct brow lift fixes drooping eyebrows, and is a fairly simple procedure. It is not the same as a forehead lift—a procedure that is done for cosmetic purposes, is expensive, and is not covered by Medicare.

If your eyelids themselves are drooping, understand that the surgery required to correct that problem is much more complicated. Talk to your eye doctor and consider your options carefully before proceeding.

────────── **MY STORY** ──────────

Seeing Better and Looking Younger

In 2001 my visual field became severely obstructed by drooping eyelids, and my doctor sent me to an ophthalmic plastic surgeon for evaluation. His diagnosis was that my eyebrows were drooping so much that they made my eyelids droop also. He took digital photos and sent them to my health insurer to see if my condition met the guidelines at that time for Medicare coverage in my state. The answer was yes, and I had a simple procedure called a "direct brow lift," in which excess skin from my forehead was removed in a wrinkle above my eyebrows. I went to a cookout the next day, wearing sunglasses that covered my eyebrows. No one was the wiser.

A few weeks after surgery, the "after" photos were compared with the photo taken before surgery. The difference was startling, and the wrinkles above my eyebrows looked no worse than they had before the surgery. There were tiny scars but, as they were right in the wrinkles, they were barely noticeable, and they faded away with time. I've retained my "younger," wide-eyed look all these years, and having a full field of vision has been helpful as my sight declines.

Improving
Reading Ability

A WELCOME SURPRISE may be in store for you if you think you can no longer read or are finding reading to be an increasingly difficult and frustrating experience. Sometimes all that is needed is properly placed, adequate lighting. Proper lighting provides the contrast that is required to distinguish the letters in words and to distinguish the type from the paper on which it is printed.

Newspapers are especially difficult to read, because they are printed on dull, grayish paper, with little contrast between the type and the paper. With macular degeneration, the light-sensing cells in the macula weaken and begin to break down as the disease progresses. This means that a greater amount of external light is needed to read. With diabetic retinopathy and macular degeneration, properly placed light is especially important, as these diseases can cause a great sensitivity to glare. To help prevent glare, position lamps so that the light is coming from above or behind you.

In this chapter, traditional ways of reading and lighting are discussed. Reading and listening on electronic devices and computer screens are discussed in Chapter 9.

Use reading stands to position material

Experiment to find the best angle and height to view reading material, holding it upright and perhaps tilting it back rather than laying it flat on a table, to make reading easier.

A reading stand is a handy way to maintain the best position of your reading material. If you usually need to move your material to the left or right to match a "good spot" in your eye, a reading stand is helpful as it allows you to move or tilt your head while keeping the reading material stationary. This may be easier for you than moving around your book or papers.

The stand in the photo, for example, can be set at four different angles and at three different heights. It holds all types of reading material, from a small book to an oversized atlas to a five-inch-wide, triple-thick three-ring binder. It is especially good for propping up a newspaper. The use of a stand also reduces arm and neck fatigue and promotes erect posture, encouraging the proper body alignment that is required for good balance. There are many other styles of reading stands, sometimes called copy holders, book holders, or book stands. Check office supply and low vision stores.

Magnifying glasses and binoculars

Sometimes magnification enlarges print enough so that you are able to read it. Magnifying glasses are available at several magnification levels, from the lowest level, 2x, up to 15x. Try different magnification levels, starting with the lowest, until you find the one that works for you. Do not

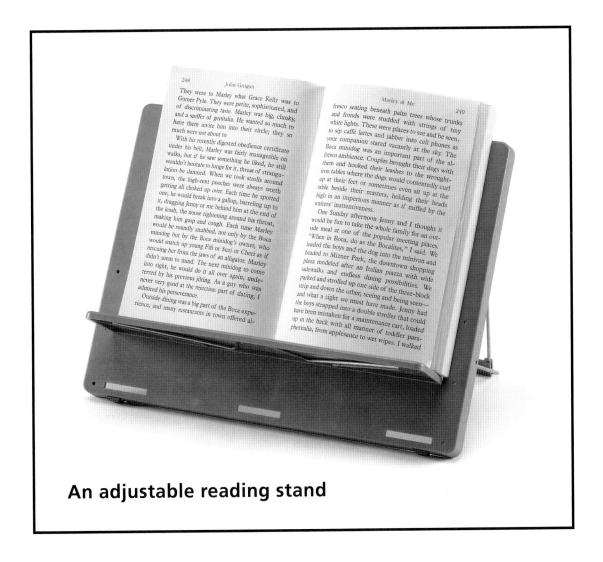

An adjustable reading stand

"buy ahead" in case you need stronger magnification later on. Get the correct strength for your current vision. Go with the minimum magnification level required, because the higher the level, the smaller the view—you see fewer letters and words as the magnification increases, even when the dimensions of the magnifiers used remain consistent.

Magnifying glasses come in various shapes, sizes, and styles. One unusual style, called a pendant, features a rectangular or round magnifier that hangs around the neck on a cord or chain, keeping the magnifier handy. Other types include pocket magnifiers, cell phone magnifiers, and magnifying mirrors.

Magnifying glasses are also available with battery-operated lights that illuminate the reading material. This is especially useful in low-light conditions. Low-priced illuminated magnifiers with LED lights come in powers ranging from 2x to 15x.

Desktop magnifiers and floor and tabletop lamps with magnifier arms are also available as described in the next section.

There are also several types of binoculars that attach to eyeglasses or to a visor. Sports spectacles have the binoculars attached to a frame. These products are good for watching sporting events, TV, and movies, and for other distance viewing tasks. Consult your low vision catalogs to see all the choices.

If you require greater magnification than is provided by magnifying glasses, consider getting one of the magnification systems that incorporate advanced technology. These systems are discussed in Chapter 9.

Choosing lamps to fit the task

For reading and close work, portable lamps—such as floor lamps, table lamps, and clip-on lights—provide good sources of direct lighting. Lamps in ceiling fixtures generally do not provide good light for reading, can produce glare, can't be aimed where you need the light to go, and it is difficult to change the bulbs. For these reasons, lighting from ceiling fixtures is not discussed further in this book.

Floor lamps with and without magnifiers

Torchiere lamps provide good general lighting that is easy on the eyes because it is indirect, with the light directed upward by a bulb in a reflecting bowl. Some models have a second, lower lamp on the pole that can give light for reading. Inexpensive models of torchiere lamps are available in chain stores.

A more substantial, and expensive, type of lamp has a magnifying lens attached, either at the light source or on a separate arm. These lamps allow your hands to remain free for reading and performing tasks. They come in both

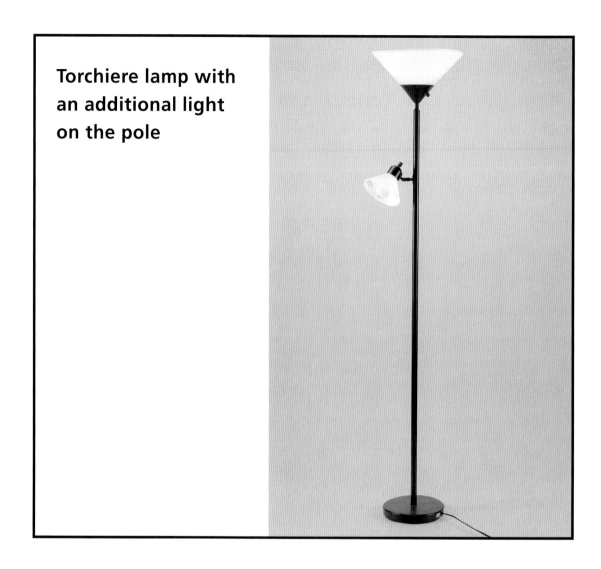

Torchiere lamp with an additional light on the pole

table and floor models, and various types accommodate incandescent, fluorescent, halogen, and "full spectrum" lightbulbs.

A Giraffe™ Lamp with a rimless magnifier on the end of an adjustable arm is shown in the photo. This lamp has a thirty-inch flexible gooseneck and a stationary anti-tip base. The height adjusts from two to seven feet. This is a particularly useful floor lamp because the long neck can easily be twisted to direct the light.

The first item I bought when my vision declined to the point that I wanted better lighting (two-and-a-half years after my diagnosis) was a Giraffe Lamp without the magnifier. I especially like this lamp because I can swing it

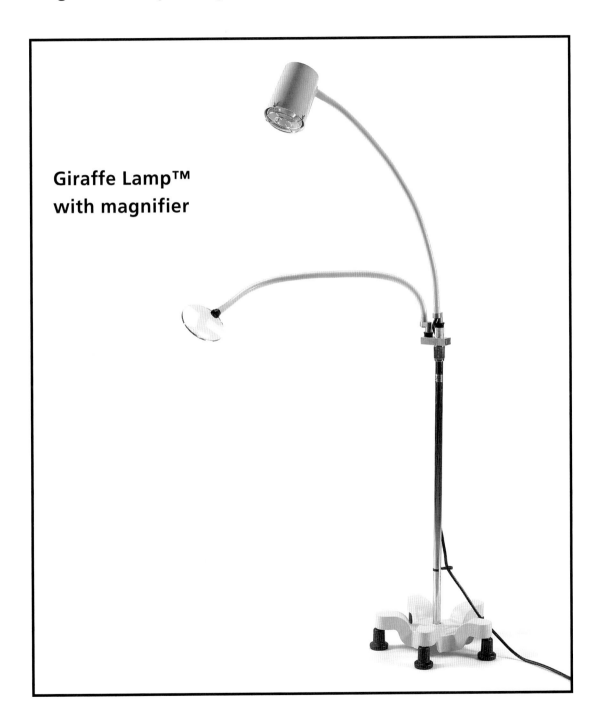

Giraffe Lamp™
with magnifier

around to where I want it in a second, and then bend it up or down as needed. As an extra bonus, the lamp swivels. Many other brands and models of lamps with magnifiers are available from low vision stores.

Desk and table lamps

Traditional table lamps with lampshades do not provide a way to direct light to where you need it to read or perform tasks such as writing checks or any other close work. When you select a lamp for a table or desk, choose one with a flexible gooseneck that can be turned to direct light where it's needed. Small lamps, like the one shown in the next photo, can be found in office supply and discount

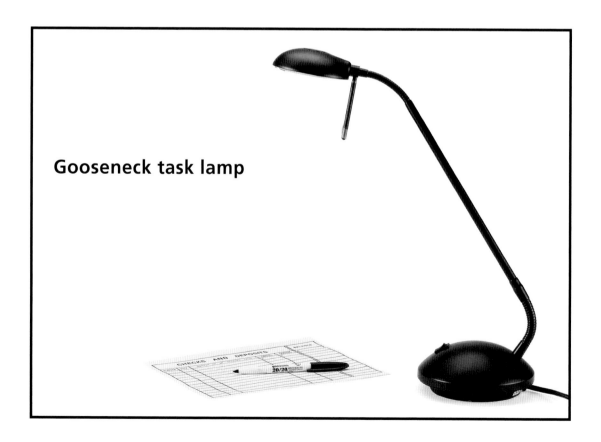

Gooseneck task lamp

stores and are reasonably priced. Look for a lamp that comes with a halogen bulb if you want really strong light. Place task lamps to your side to avoid reflected glare from your work surface. Avoid looking directly at a bare bulb that is turned on.

For even brighter task lighting, you may consider a magnifying desk lamp. This type of lamp has a high-

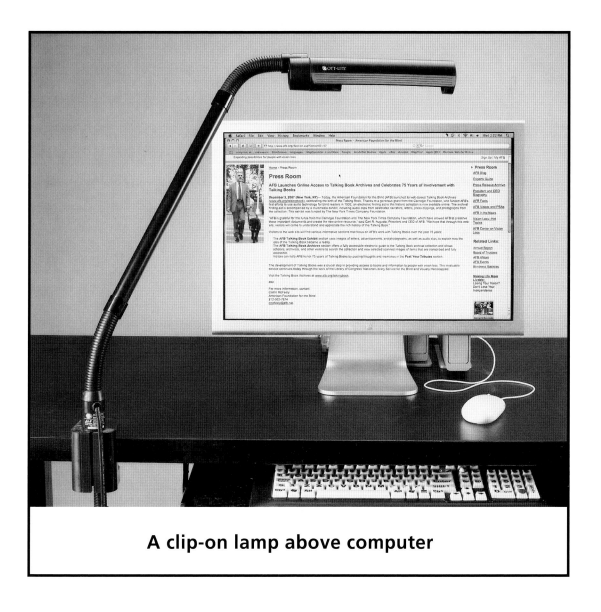

A clip-on lamp above computer

intensity bulb and powerful magnification. These lamps cost less than the magnifying floor models.

Clip-on lamps are useful for attaching a light source to a desk, a computer stand, or the headboard of a bed. These lamps are widely available in discount and home center stores.

Spot lighting

When you need to aim light at a particular spot, use a small lamp that directs the light right at the object you want to see. I use a small clip-on lamp above my microwave oven, positioned so that it shines light on the oven's buttons. When I first bought this oven, I could easily read the buttons' white numbers on the black background, but after a couple of years I could no longer detect them—the entire control panel appeared black. The small light allows me to easily see the numbers once again.

Flashlights

Perhaps the most indispensable type of light is the flashlight. One type of small handy flashlight is the pen light. You can direct the light at a line of text, such as on a menu or in a book. These lights come in models with bright LED bulbs. The small flashlights shown in the photo can stand up because they have been placed in a device called the Flashlite Friend™. This tool also allows the flashlight to point downward—a useful position for aiming light at a menu or a plate in a dark restaurant. Servers are always fascinated by the way the flashlight can stand in so many positions. The small, six-inch flashlights shown here have also been wrapped in reflective tape to make them easy to spot, even in the dark.

It is a good idea to have several flashlights, each in a Flashlite Friend, available so you can find one when you need it. When placing flashlights around the house, stand them on end so they are easier to find in the dark. This is especially handy when you need to find a light quickly during a power outage. When you are going out, you can

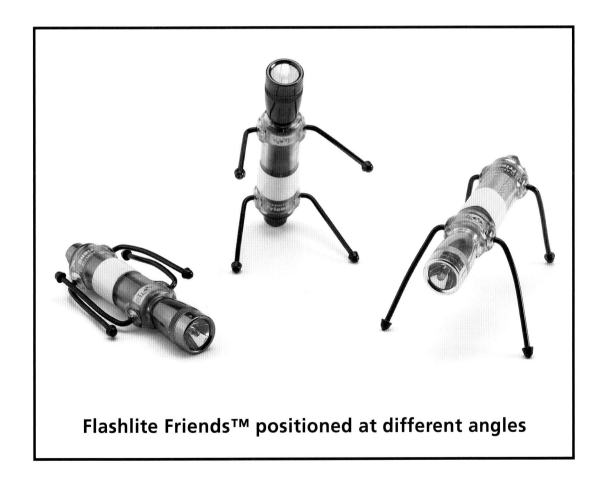

Flashlite Friends™ positioned at different angles

fold the legs of the Flashlite Friend and bring it with you. Always carry a flashlight so that you're not accidentally left without one when you're away from home.

Handy places to keep flashlights

- In the car—a must
- In the kitchen, to help find things in the refrigerator and in cupboards
- By your bed, to help you when you get up at night
- In your purse, briefcase, or pocket—indispensable at dimly lit restaurants, for reading the menu and, propped up, for seeing your food
- By thermostats, if you need to adjust the settings
- By chairs and tables, so that you can find things that fall
- On your bureau, to help you see contents of drawers and locate items

Never leave home without a flashlight!

Lantern-style flashlights for power outages

Lantern-style flashlights provide strong lighting during power outages. Three models are shown here. They each have a handle that makes them easy to carry; but even so, it is a good idea to have two or three lanterns that you can place in various rooms in the event of a power outage. Find a special place to keep the lanterns when they're not in use so that they are easily accessible in the dark. I have three lanterns of different styles, and I keep them on top of the refrigerator because I know I can always find an object that large, even in the dark. I position each of my lanterns with the handle facing outward so I don't have to grapple in the dark to pick one up.

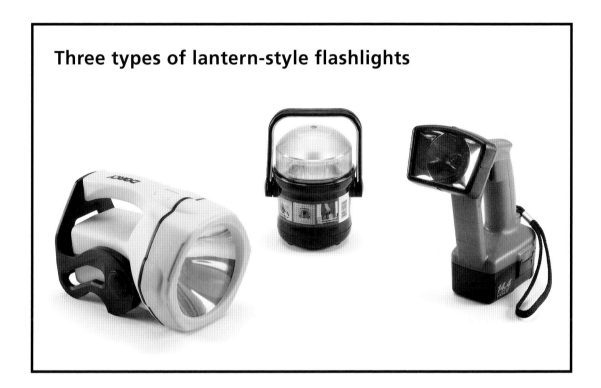

Three types of lantern-style flashlights

Night-lights

Although they are not for reading, night-lights are indispensable for helping you find your way in the dark. Put one in your bedroom, bathroom, hallways, and any other areas where you are likely to walk at night. Also, have a beacon by your bed, such as a lighted clock on a bedside table.

Choosing the best type of lightbulb for your current needs

Selecting lightbulbs can be a confusing experience because there are so many types and sizes. The following descriptions may help you select the type that is best for your needs.

- **Incandescent.** This is the type of bulb you probably grew up with. It is a reliable light source, but it is not energy efficient and it burns out more quickly than newer types, so you must change the bulbs often. The government has mandated that the manufacturing of these bulbs is to be discontinued in favor of more energy-efficient alternatives.

- **Compact fluorescent.** These bulbs are available in many shapes and sizes that screw into regular sockets. Though more expensive than incandescent bulbs, they last much longer and more than pay for themselves in energy savings. They come in warm, cool, and full-spectrum colors, and they do not have the annoying flutter that long fluorescent tubes sometimes have.

- **Halogen.** This type of bulb is useful for track and task lighting. Halogen bulbs come in a variety of sizes and shapes, with bulbs for track lighting available in angles from 13 to 60 degrees. As my vision has declined, I have moved to the 40-degree bulbs, because the larger angle covers more territory.

- **Natural daylight or full spectrum.** These bulbs provide light that simulates natural daylight. Many people who are troubled by glare find these bulbs restful. They are available both as incandescent and compact fluorescent bulbs.

- **LED (Light Emitting Diode).** In addition to their original use in flashlights, LED lighting is available in desk and task lamps.

As your vision changes over time, experiment with different types of bulbs in your various lamps. In the early stages of your disease you may not even need special lighting, as was my case for more than two years. As time passes, keep trying different bulbs until you find the best type for each particular lamp and location. Realize that your needs can keep changing, so keep trying until you find the best lamp-bulb combination for you at that particular time. Remember that what works well for you now may not work well for you in the future, so keep experimenting over the years to see if a different bulb might allow you to see more clearly.

—————— MY STORY ——————

Glare Led Me to Switch Types of Bulbs

Another symptom of the problem in my right eye was a sudden sensitivity to glare. I could no longer read in the dining room, where I had always read the newspaper. My dining room has two light sources—a Giraffe Lamp and an overhead fixture. Fortunately, I keep a supply of four different kinds of bulbs—incandescent, compact fluorescent, full spectrum, and halogen. When I found the glare in the dining room overpowering, I replaced the halogen bulb in the Giraffe Lamp with a full-spectrum bulb, and the incandescent bulb in the ceiling fixture with a compact fluorescent bulb. Now I am again comfortable reading in that room, and if my needs change I will again try different combinations of bulbs.

Nurturing Your Body

YOU HAVE MANY SENSES in addition to eyesight, and this is the time to start fine-tuning them. In addition to the five commonly known senses of sight, hearing, taste, touch, and smell, there are two others that are especially important to people with vision loss. The first is the perception of balance. The second is the perception of your own body—the awareness of your posture and positioning and feelings of movements of your body. These are senses that people are frequently not aware of, but rely on enormously.

Develop your sensory systems now because they become more and more important as time goes on. And while you are at it, work on improving your general physical well-being and fitness level.

Guidelines for a healthy lifestyle

The eye, like any other part of the body, benefits from a healthful diet. Suggested guidelines for a healthy lifestyle from the National Eye Institute of the U.S. National Institutes of Health and from retinologists are listed here. The recommendations are important for everyone, but they are particularly important for anyone who has a macular disease, as well as for his or her children and grandchildren, as macular diseases frequently have genetic components. In my own case, my mother, uncle, and a first cousin all developed a macular disease, and we've traced it back to the maternal side of my mother's family. Your entire family would benefit from following these suggestions.

- Exercise and increase physical activity.

- Eat a healthful diet high in fruits, green leafy vegetables (especially kale and spinach for macular degeneration), and fish.

- Watch your weight and reduce your fat intake.

- Maintain normal blood pressure and cholesterol levels.

- Do not smoke.

- If you have diabetes, it is important to control your levels of blood sugar, blood pressure, and blood cholesterol. Doing so can help prevent the development and progression of diabetic retinopathy.

Doctors recommend that your adult children have annual eye examinations, even if they do not require eyeglasses, starting at age fifty; and at the appointment, tell the doctor about the family history of macular disease.

Exercise to develop your senses of balance and body awareness

Exercise becomes more important as vision decreases. We don't realize how much we rely on looking ahead at objects to anchor ourselves in the space we occupy, so it is important to develop inner balance and body awareness. During exercise, the brain and muscles learn to communicate more efficiently. Exercise helps build confidence in the way your body moves. Being active helps ensure that you can maintain your independence, including your ability to do daily activities such as grooming, bathing, dressing, preparing food, and walking. Motivating yourself to start exercising can be difficult, but physical activity is crucial to nurturing your body. You do not need to excel at sports to gain from and enjoy exercise, and you can start at any age and still receive great benefits.

Exercise for independence

Before starting an exercise program, make an appointment with your doctor, who may offer suggestions on specific types of exercise from among the types listed below.

■ Aerobic exercise to improve cardiovascular fitness, immune function, cognitive function, and mood

■ Strength training to build and maintain muscle and bone mass

- Flexibility training to improve motion throughout each body joint
- Balance training to prevent falls and develop confident movement

Although each type of exercise is important, balance training is especially critical for someone with vision loss because of the danger of falling when it is difficult to see your surroundings. Follow the suggestions below when developing your general fitness program.

- Consult health professionals, such as physical and occupational therapists, for a determination of your strengths and areas of deficit.
- Add their recommendations for balance training to your exercise program.
- Join a class that includes balance exercises.
- Work to develop a good internal sense of balance and the ability to quickly right yourself when thrown off balance.
- Wear shoes with good fit and support and with soles that prevent slipping, but that don't excessively grip the floor.
- Remember that when you are tired, stressed, or distracted, you may respond poorly to challenges, so take extra care.
- Get adequate rest, because it helps ensure quick responses by body and mind.

- Learn exercises and do them in short periods of five to ten minutes throughout the day—you'll benefit just as much from these short separate sessions as you would from one long session.

Find a class to support your exercise program

After consulting a healthcare professional, it is a good idea to join a class to stay motivated and to receive instruction on how to properly perform exercises. Classes are offered in community recreation centers, community education programs, senior centers, churches, and low vision organizations. If you belong to a health club, you can get individual instruction from a trainer, who can design a program for you.

You might find it helpful to attend classes in yoga, Pilates, and/or tai chi. Tai chi is especially helpful because it helps to develop inner balance without relying on focusing on a spot in the distance, which you are probably now doing to anchor yourself when doing balance exercises. Choosing physical activities that you enjoy encourages you to practice consistently at home to gain optimal benefits.

If you are not physically able to take a class or do standing exercises at home, you can do chair exercises sitting right in your own living room. Most states have a service that provides a closed-circuit radio network with special programming for those who are unable to read or hold reading material. An exercise program is often included in the service's scheduled programming.

My mother faithfully did her chair exercises even though she had severe arthritis and only peripheral vision. These sessions helped her keep a positive attitude and seemed to make her feel better. You can find a radio station in your area by checking the International Association of Audio Information Services' website at http://iaais.org/locateservice.html or by calling your state's department of services for the blind. You can also listen to broadcasts of these radio programs on the Internet. See page 206 for more information on these radio services. Also, sometimes public and community television stations offer exercise programming.

Consider that strength and agility are needed for driving

There is another motivation to start exercising. Most people want to keep driving as long as possible, but often we believe good vision is all that is required. Stop to think about all the muscle groups you use when you drive, and you can understand how exercise can help keep you behind the wheel.

Just to get into the car you need strong leg and upper body muscles. Once you start to drive, you use foot, ankle, and calf muscles for braking and accelerating. Your arms, wrists, and fingers are needed for steering and using dashboard controls. You must have agility to be a safe driver. Your neck must be flexible and strong to be able to turn to check blind spots when changing lanes. Torso strength and agility are needed so that you can twist to the left and right to see what is behind you when preparing to back up. Ankles must be flexible to push the pedals. Driving is definitely a full-body activity.

See Chapter 10 for a more detailed discussion of driving.

MY STORY

An Athletic Failure,
But a Lover of Exercise

As a child, teenager, and college student, I tried one sport after the other, both in school gym class and at neighborhood ball games. No matter whether it was softball, basketball, volleyball, swimming, or, finally, golf—I was the last person wanted on any team. I totally lacked whatever it is that makes one able to perform at even a minimum level in sports.

Then, in my early twenties, I discovered an adult beginners' ballet class and found the joy of dance. Although not innately talented, I was able to do the classic exercises at the barre, and I advanced to work in the center of the room where there was nothing to hold on to. I continued classes for a few years, then stopped until my late forties, when I found another adult beginners' class. My love of balletic exercise was renewed, and I took classes for another couple of years.

Thirty years passed until I found a ballet class for mature adults offered through my community's adult education program. By then I was seventy-four years old, and my body had forgotten everything it had once known about ballet. My teachers, a husband-and-wife team, were tolerant, and they welcomed me into their beginning and intermediate classes.

Through another lucky connection, I discovered Pilates, a mind-body exercise system with an approach to movement that emphasizes body alignment, breathing, strength, flexibility, balance, and endurance. My instructor, who is also an occupational therapist, knew exactly how to help me develop the strength and balance I needed to move forward with my study of ballet.

I was still missing strength and aerobic training components, and at the age of eighty, I added kettlebells (a cast iron weight that looks like a bowling ball with a handle on top) to my program. These exercise activities bring me a feeling of exhilaration, and they have given me a level of fitness that has helped me through some trying times. I need the sustenance of body and spirit that exercise provides.

Develop your sense of touch

Start thinking about your sense of touch, which you may have been taking for granted. Touch becomes more important as vision decreases because touch can help compensate for diminished sight. You feel through nerve endings that act as touch receptors through your skin. Your fingertips are especially sensitive because they have more receptors than most other parts of the body. Just think about how much a small paper cut on the tip of your finger hurts.

This sensitivity allows you to feel the difference between rough and smooth, soft and hard, hot and cold, and wet and dry. Feeling an object tells you if it is flat or raised, round or square. Later chapters describe how your sense of touch is important in the kitchen and in finding hard-to-spot things that have been identified with special marks.

Find pleasure in feeling various textures and objects

Some items that give sensory pleasure when touched or stroked are fabrics such as fleece or velvet, rocks, smooth or textured glass, and wood or metal objects such as sculptures. Petting your cat or dog gives pleasure to both you and your pet. Hugs are felt through your skin, and they can make you feel good all over and can reduce stress. Look for things you enjoy feeling and touching, to enjoy now—and later.

Practice identifying objects by feel and shape

As you go about your daily activities, become aware of the shapes and sizes of objects you use throughout the day. When you put away dishes, for instance, you can tell the difference between large and small plates and bowls and short and tall glasses. This enables you to put things in their designated places in your cupboards even if it's difficult to see where they belong. You can learn to tell the difference between knives, forks, and spoons by their shapes and weights. I remember family celebrations and watching my mother and her blind brother, my Uncle Matt, put away silverware after the feast. I can hear her now, saying, "You can tell the good silverware by its heft and weight. Keep it separate from the everyday knives and forks."

Optimize your sense of hearing

As sight diminishes, hearing becomes more and more important. We may not realize how frequently we use our hearing in many areas of our lives, such as when driving—a strong motivation to have your hearing tested if you suspect a hearing loss. As your sight diminishes, good hearing helps you to connect with other people and listen to books and other printed material that have been recorded in audio form.

Get your hearing checked

It is best to have your hearing checked by a licensed audiologist to ensure that you receive a thorough examination. If you go to an ear doctor for an examination, the doctor can probably refer you to an audiologist if you need a hearing aid. Simply responding to an ad you receive in the mail for a "free hearing evaluation" may not result in the comprehensive evaluation you require. Medicare covers the costs of hearing tests, so you can have your hearing tested by a reputable, licensed audiologist. Entrust your hearing only to a qualified professional.

Licensed audiologists may work in private practices or in hospitals or clinics. If there are underlying medical issues that are causing your hearing to be affected, your audiologist may refer you to an ENT (ear, nose, and throat) physician, also called an otolaryngologist. If your hearing tests show that you would be helped by a hearing aid, the audiologist can discuss a variety of hearing aid choices with you.

If you have a hearing loss, you will greatly benefit from using hearing aids. Unfortunately, they are expensive, and they are not covered by Medicare. Some health insurance plans pay a portion of the cost, but usually not every year—every three years is a common period. If the price is out of your reach, discuss your situation with your audiologist—sometimes arrangements can be made for a manufacturer or other source to help you with the expense.

Changing hearing aid batteries

Use of a hearing aid involves the sense of touch. It requires good finger dexterity to insert a hearing aid in your ear. Although removal is easier, it still requires dexterity. It is quite possible to accidentally drop an aid on the floor. A bigger challenge is handling the batteries.

My first two hearing aids were "completely in the canal" models that use number-10 batteries. I got the first aid, for my left ear, in 1996—long before I had any vision loss. Handling the tiny batteries was no problem until my vision decreased and I could barely see where to put in a new battery. I tried changing a battery with my eyes closed, but was not successful. Even with my eyes open, I was dropping the tiny batteries on the floor. Eventually I learned to change batteries over a counter or table to minimize the danger of them falling. Sitting in an upholstered chair to change a battery can lead to the battery falling into a cranny of the chair, making it even harder to find than one that has landed on the floor.

Dropped or lost batteries can be more than an aggravation in trying to find them—they can be dangerous to a pet or a young grandchild, who might be attracted to them and swallow them. Even though hearing aid batteries no longer contain mercury and do not need to be recycled, they can cause serious gastric problems if swallowed.

I now have large, behind-the-ear hearing aids for both ears. They use the large, number-13 battery. My audiologist picked out the brand of aid that was easiest in terms of changing batteries. I practiced changing the battery with my eyes closed several times, and I was successful.

At the time I began using the first aid with the number-13 battery, my hearing was still at a level that would have allowed me to continue using another small hearing aid that required number-10 batteries, but I wanted to be prepared for both future hearing loss and the need to manipulate the batteries with diminished vision. My aids

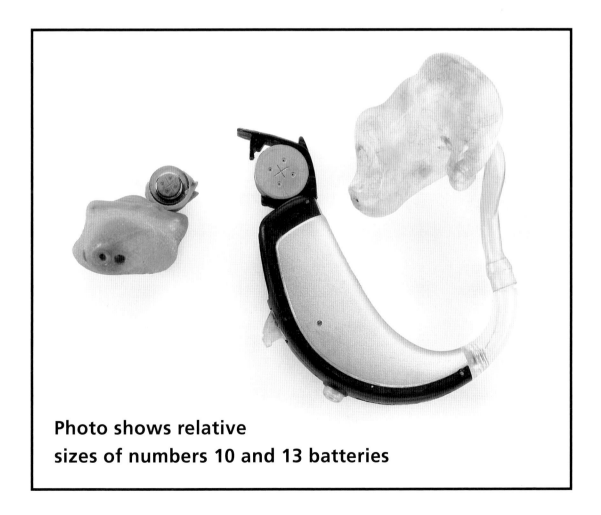

Photo shows relative
sizes of numbers 10 and 13 batteries

are currently set at about the middle volume level, and the audiologist can program the volume to higher levels as time goes on.

Are you lip reading without realizing it?

I was surprised when my audiologist had me perform tests that showed I was relying heavily on lip reading without even realizing it. First she placed me in a booth with a glass wall dividing us. I was wearing special earphones that allowed me to hear her voice, and I could see her on the other side of the glass wall as she read word after word. As she said each word, I tried to repeat it out loud back to her. She kept a score of how many I got correct. Then I closed my eyes so that I could not see her enunciating the words. I was amazed to learn that I got ninety-two percent of the words correct when I was watching the audiologist, but only seventy-two percent correct when I could not see her. These results showed that I was doing a lot of lip reading.

Here are some helpful strategies for dealing with a hearing loss when you also have diminished vision. These ideas were suggested to me by my audiologist, and I have found them quite useful.

- Train yourself to listen—try closing your eyes when watching television or chatting with someone, or listen to an audio book.
- Ask people to speak slowly and enunciate clearly.

- Ask people to look directly at you when speaking so that the sound comes directly to you. Even if you can't watch their lips, you may be able to see their body language and gestures, such as arm waving—valuable cues that help you understand what the speakers are saying.

- Find the best listening spot in your house of worship by trying different seating locations.

- Use assistive listening devices at movies, theaters, concerts, and other such venues.

- Use a personal amplifier when watching TV.

- In restaurants, ask for a quiet table off to the side, near a wall. Face the wall rather than the room—if you sit facing the room, with all the noise in front of you and a quiet wall behind you, the speaker's voice at your table can become overpowered by all the noise that is also coming right at you from the room. When you face the wall, the loudest sounds come from the people speaking at your table who are facing you.

Most important of all—be an advocate for yourself and let others know what you need.

MY STORY

The Dog Ate My Hearing Aid

Be careful where you put your hearing aids. Even more dangerous to a pet than swallowing a battery is eating an entire hearing aid. If you have a pet, be careful to place your aids in their containers when you remove them from your ears. Dogs and cats are attracted to the hum of a hearing aid that hasn't been turned off, as well as to the scent of wax that may adhere to the inner part of a hearing aid.

When I still had the small aid, I carelessly placed my aid on my bedside table for an afternoon rest. That night, my son's visiting dog became violently ill. I didn't make the connection until a couple of days later, when I realized my aid was hopelessly lost. Fortunately the hearing aid was very small and the dog recovered, but a larger aid could have caused serious internal injuries.

Things turned out just fine for the dog, but I had to spend hundreds of dollars on a new hearing aid.

Use talking healthcare products that announce your results

There is a huge variety of specialty products that provide audio as well as visual information. These products can help you remain independent in taking care of personal healthcare tasks. They are available at low vision stores. Here are just some of the "talking" products available.

- Blood pressure monitors
- Glucose meters

- Pedometers that announce the numbers of steps you have taken and the total distance traveled

- Scales that speak your weight or that have detachable displays that you can hold as close to your eyes as you need in order to read them

- Thermometers that state your temperature reading

Use special products and tricks in personal care

The ideas listed below are helpful as you go about your tasks of personal care.

Brushing teeth— hazards and solutions

- Use an electric toothbrush that is kept upright in a stand on your vanity and can stand upright on your counter in between charging. You'll be able to find the toothbrush easily, and electric toothbrushes help you to take good care of your teeth.

- Toothpaste in a pump dispenser that stands upright on the counter is easier to find than a tube that can easily disappear when you put it down on your bathroom vanity.

- Match up the toothpaste squirting out of the dispenser with the bristles of the toothbrush by putting the toothpaste on your finger, then transferring it to the toothbrush—or, even easier, put the toothpaste on your finger, then transfer it directly to your mouth.

■ I learned a good trick the hard way when friends in ballet class and other places told me I had toothpaste around my mouth and even on my cheek. I can no longer see in the mirror well enough to know that I'm not "clean." Now I always splash water all over my face, or even better, wipe with a wet washcloth. As a final check, I feel around my mouth with my finger and if I find a sticky spot, it's probably toothpaste I've missed.

Caring for nails

■ Use emery boards instead of nail clippers to keep fingernails and toenails trimmed—you can file by feel, and you won't accidentally cut too much or injure yourself.

■ Have a regular pedicure if basic toenail care is difficult for you. Note that home visits by pedicurists are available in some communities, and many senior centers offer the services of visiting pedicurists or nurses. If you would rather not visit a pedicurist for basic toenail maintenance but you have a hard time reaching your toes, try to enlist the help of a friend or relative who will keep your toenails in good condition by filing them with an emery board.

■ Visit a podiatrist for nail clipping and to care for foot problems such as ingrown toenails or other foot-related problems such as corns or calluses. If you are diabetic, this service is likely to be covered by Medicare.

Grooming

- Lipstick can be difficult to apply properly, so instead try tinted lip gloss. If you "go outside the lines," it is not noticeable. Lip glosses usually cost less than lipstick, and some brands also act as moisturizing lip balms.

- Use magnifying mirrors for close-work grooming tasks. These are available in many sizes, shapes, and magnification levels. Some are lighted. There are handheld models, models on stands, and wall-mounted models with the magnifiers at the end of swivel arms.

- Use an electric razor for shaving safety.

Bathing and showering

- Install grab bars in your tub and shower areas. They help you orient yourself in the shower and provide a means of support when getting in and out of the shower or tub. For more information on grab bars, see pages 100–101.

- Use a shower bench or transfer bench if you feel unsteady in the shower or if you find it difficult to enter or exit the tub or shower. For photos and more information on these products, see pages 100–102.

PART 2

Using Practical Hints to Make Your Life Easier

IDEAS FOR INDEPENDENT day-to-day living are offered in this section. Some involve using or rearranging things you already have, while others involve low-cost products designed for people with vision loss. These products are available at low vision stores, which carry a huge variety of other useful items as well. Most of the products described in this book are available from one or more of the stores that are listed in Appendix B, Suppliers of Low Vision Products. There is space in this book to discuss only a small portion of the many useful products that can be purchased, but most of the stores listed offer catalogs that you can order, either over the phone or by visiting store websites. Order your catalogs today!

Cooking and Eating Use Senses of Touch and Hearing

WOULD YOU GUESS that your sense of touch could become the most important sense when cooking? You might first think of taste, then smell. You may be surprised by how important your sense of touch is in compensating for a diminishing sense of sight. Even your sense of hearing becomes important in the kitchen.

As you go about your tasks in the kitchen, be aware of activities that are becoming difficult and start thinking about new ways to do them. Develop the attitude of a creative thinker who is finding solutions to cooking challenges. The ideas suggested here can start you along that path. Some of the ideas in this food section are my own, but most were learned in an inspiring class I took at Vision Loss Resources in Minneapolis. The name of the class is Independent Living Skills, and the methods taught have been gathered from participants over an eighteen-year period. I am indebted to everyone who shared their ideas over the years.

Prepare food more easily with useful items

Use these simple items as you learn the new ways to cook.

- Set of metal measuring cups with raised dots
- Two sets of metal measuring spoons with raised dots; the spoons of one set bent at right angles to make dippers
- Special paint pens that make permanent raised dots to identify items
- Saucer
- Funnels of various sizes
- Needle-nose pliers or ring opener
- Timer with large numbers that talks or has loud ring
- Towels—one dark, one white
- Cutting boards—one black, one white—or various colors
- Heavy rubber bands
- Pair of fingered gloves with nonslip silicone grips

Using your sense of touch in the kitchen

People with diminished vision often have difficulty identifying items such as measuring cups and spoons or dials on the stove and oven. A solution is to use a special paint pen to apply small dots of paint that raise, harden, and become waterproof and dishwasher-proof. These dots are informally known as "high marks." You can develop your sense of touch by feeling the number of dots on the handles and dials on your appliances.

Paint pens are available at low vision stores. They come in a variety of colors, including black, white, and orange, and the paint adheres to just about any surface, including plastic and metal. One brand of tactile paint pen is the

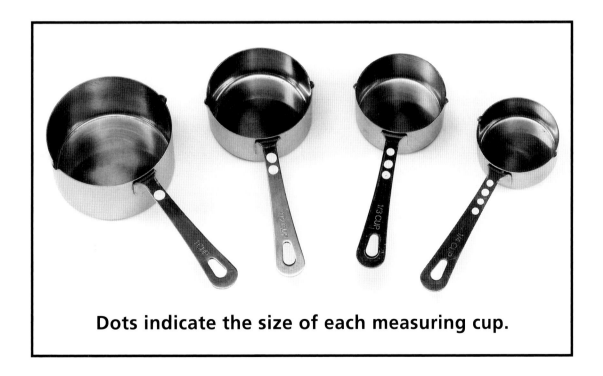

Dots indicate the size of each measuring cup.

HI-MARK™. The dots are produced by squirting a paint-like substance from the pen onto the surface you want to mark.

In order to make sure there is plenty of space for placing the dots, get metal measuring cups and spoons with long handles. Place the dots on the handles close to the cup or spoon so you are able to grasp the handles and slide your thumb along the top of the handle to feel the number of dots. To tell one measuring cup from another, put one dot on the 1-cup measure, two dots on the ½-cup measure,

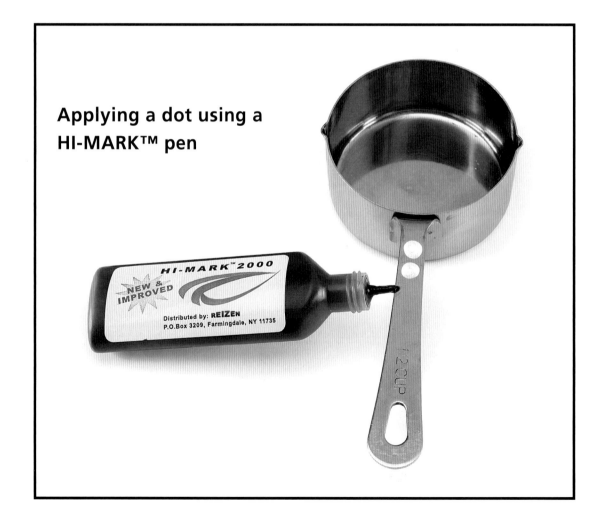

Applying a dot using a HI-MARK™ pen

three dots on the ⅓-cup measure, and four dots on the ¼-cup measure. Use the same system with your measuring spoons.

Stoves and ovens—electric or gas?

Burners on electric ranges and stoves are generally safer than gas burners because it is easier to see the color of the coils of an electric burner (which becomes redder as it becomes hotter) than it is to see any height of the blue flame on a gas burner. Even a flashlight beam pointed at a gas burner does not make its flame visible, so it can be impossible to tell, just by looking, whether a low flame is still going or if it is extinguished. A suggestion is to apply high marks on the dial at the settings you generally use. Newer stoves and ovens have touchpad technology instead of knobs. Pressing on the appropriate textured region activates a control that results in a clearly audible beep tone. It helps to use high marks or bumps to indicate your favorite settings.

Another idea is to buy an electric skillet. The model I have has a separate heat control that plugs into the skillet. The control has a dial similar to that of an oven's temperature heat-setting dial, but with a top temperature of 400 degrees.

No matter the heat source, it is wise to cook over low and medium heat, as you don't want to take chances with a high heat that could lead to boilovers or scorches.

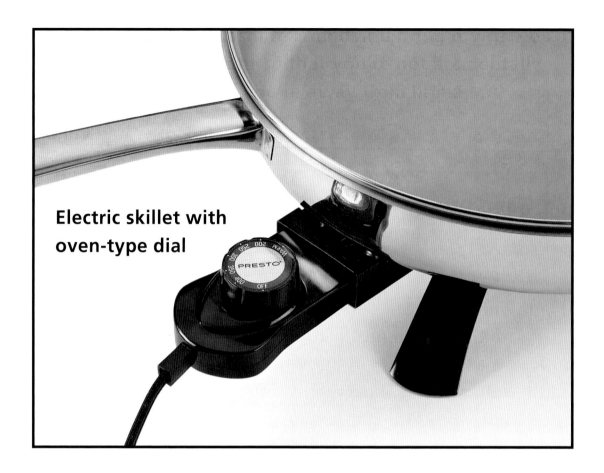

Electric skillet with oven-type dial

For ovens, it is a good idea to place a high mark at the 350-degree setting so it is easy to find.

Microwave cooking

Follow these useful tips when using your microwave oven.

■ Use your sense of hearing: listen closely to the number of beeps when you press the buttons to set the cooking time. One extra push of the minute button, for instance, could lead to overcooking, a smoke-filled oven, or worse.

- Buy frozen vegetables in bags rather than in boxes and remove just the portion you want, then close the bag and put it back in your freezer for the next use.

- Cook bacon in the microwave oven by placing strips between several sheets of paper towels to make thick pads to absorb the fat.

When selecting a new microwave oven, consider looking for a model with some of the following special options.

- With a "30 seconds" button, you can easily set the time for ½, 1½, or 2½ minutes.

- Use contrasting display colors, such as black print on a white background or white print on a black background. Find the color combination that is easiest for you to see.

- A "talking" feature can prompt you to set the time and announce cooking time settings, the running cooking time, the current power level, and such phrases as "microwave running," "attend to food," and so forth. High-end models that announce the current time and that have a speech volume control are available at low vision stores.

- A sensor helps to prevent overcooking or undercooking by determining when the food is ready based on infrared light or by the steam emitted from the food.

- Choose the door handle that works best for you, whether it requires pulling or has a bar or button to push to open the door.

For a review of the accessibility and reviews of microwave ovens and other kitchen and laundry appliances, visit the American Foundation for the Blind's website and enter "Appliances" in the search box. (www.afb.org)

Following recipes

Always start by washing your hands—because you will use your fingers in new ways. When making something in a mixing bowl, first lay out all your ingredients to one side of the bowl. After each ingredient is added, move its container to the other side of the bowl. Then you do not have to wonder whether you have added a particular item. For contrast and to catch spills, place a dark towel underneath a white bowl and a white towel under a dark bowl.

Measuring ingredients

Your sense of touch again comes into play when using measuring cups and spoons. First place a towel on your work space to catch drips and spills and to keep bowls and cutting boards from sliding.

If you are working with wet ingredients, keep a saucer handy as a place to put measuring cups and spoons that may be dripping. If you are measuring dry ingredients such as flour or sugar, find the size of measure you want and dip it into the canister. But don't use a knife to level the scoopful. You have a much handier instrument—your index finger.

For small amounts of wet and liquid ingredients, use measuring spoons that have been bent to form dippers. If you are unable to see how much of an ingredient is in a measuring spoon, use your finger to feel off the top.

Using a knife on a cutting board

The safe way to find the sharp side of a knife is with your sense of touch. Grasp the handle and use your index finger to feel the notch at the end. The side with the notch is the sharp side, so turn the knife so that side is on the bottom. To provide contrast, use a black or dark cutting board to slice light foods, such as onions, and a white cutting board to slice dark foods, such as cooked meat. Silicone cutting boards come in a variety of bright colors.

Cooking on the range or stovetop

Here are some handy tips on using senses other than sight to prepare foods on stovetops.

- Rolling boils can be detected in two ways—by hearing the boil or by using your hand, placed a few inches above the pan, to feel the amount of steam being produced.

- Judge whether or not onions have become golden brown by sampling some that have cooled a bit. Both the taste of the onion and its tender texture lets you know.

- When frying foods, place a splatter guard on top of the pan. The guard prevents hot grease and little pieces of food from flying out of the pan to those hard-to-spot, hard-to-clean places on your stove.

Cooking in the oven

Follow these handy tips when cooking food in the oven.

- Pour cake batter into just one spot in the pan (even a Bundt pan), then level off, first by quickly sliding the pan on the counter, first from side to side, then away from and toward you. Finish off the process with a couple of taps of the pan on the counter.

- Never reach into a hot or heating oven to place a pan on the rack or to remove the pan from the rack. Instead, wear your oven-safe gloves, pull out the rack, and place or remove your pan. This safety measure prevents burns.

Using timers

Many types of timers are available from low vision stores. Timers range in size from small digital models that are about three inches in height to a dial model that is a huge nine inches in diameter and has a loud and long ring. There are also timers you can hang around your neck. Research the possibilities and choose a model that seems right for you. You may want to try a few different types. Set the timer for the amount of time a food is to be cooked or when it is to be checked, and (use your sense of hearing) listen for the ring that tells you the set amount of time has elapsed. Timers don't have to be used just for cooking—you may want to also keep some in other rooms, such as your bedroom to awaken you from a nap.

Pouring liquids into a glass or cup

- For dark liquids such as coffee, use a cup that is white on the inside to provide contrast.

- For white liquids, use a colored glass or one with a pattern. Water can be difficult to see in any type of glass because it is transparent.

Managing coffee making

I enjoy a couple of cups of coffee when I get up in the morning, and have developed some useful tricks that avoid several possible hazards. My first step was to get a 12- × 16-inch plastic tray with a lip all the way around. These are available at discount stores, and they come in a variety of bright colors. Place all the items you need on the tray:

Coffeemaker
Coffee can
Funnels
Cups
Straws

Now follow these steps.

- Fill the carafe to the level for the number of cups you want. See pages 107–108 for instruction on making the lines easier to see.

- Use a funnel when you can't see the hole for pouring the water into the coffeemaker, and slowly pour the water into the funnel—with no splashes or spills.

- Put the desired number of scoops into the basket. To check the level of coffee in the scoop, hold it with one hand and feel the top with your index finger, leveling off if necessary.

- When pouring the coffee, I often pour over the top of my morning coffee cup—a situation requiring acceptance of my vision loss and patience with myself—but my spills are limited to the tray and I don't end up with coffee all over the counter and dripping down on the floor.

- If you pour over the top and the coffee overflows, do not attempt to pick up the cup. Put a straw into the coffee cup and sip enough coffee to make it safe to pick up the cup.

- To see the cup on the dark table, I put my cup on a white paper napkin to make it visible. This is safer than a coaster that is raised above the table and easier to tip. I haven't broken a cup yet!

Tray with coffee maker with funnel, coffee can, cup, and straws

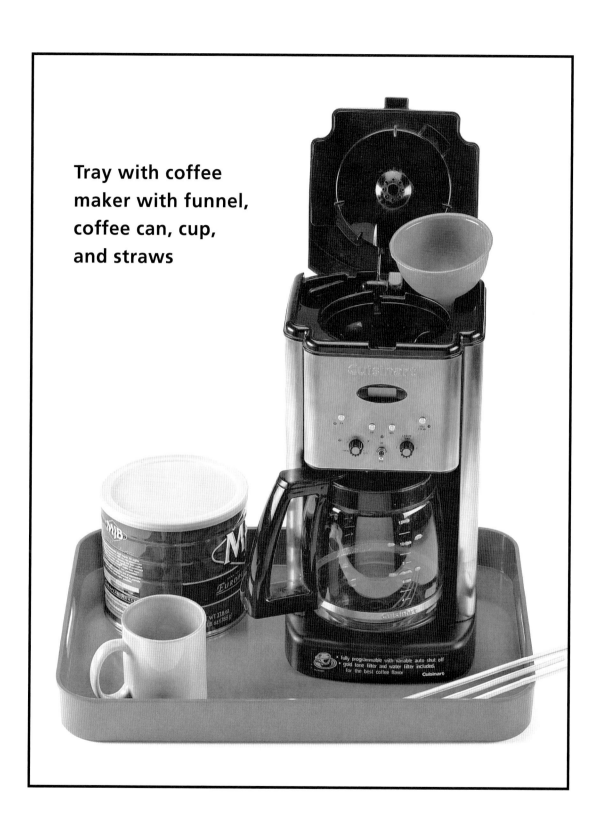

More tricks of the trade from cooks who would not give up

- You can measure out one tablespoon from a stick of butter by using your index finger as a measure, placing it flat, perpendicular to the length of the butter.

- It is very difficult to feel most oils at room temperature, and most cooking oils solidify when kept in the refrigerator. Canola oil (one of the more healthful oils) is the only oil that remains a liquid when stored in the refrigerator. When pouring it into a glass or cup, you are able to feel the level of the chilled liquid.

- Spray the inside of measuring cups with vegetable oil spray so food doesn't stick to the cups.

- Use oil sprays over the sink so you don't get any on the floor and slip.

- Marinate meat in a zipped plastic bag.

- Find which side of a milk carton to open by sliding your finger along the top to feel which side has the crease.

- To open cans with pull tabs, use needle-nose pliers or just stick a spoon under the tab.

Use large print and specialty cookbooks

Many cookbooks are available in large print versions that are easier to read than regular editions. You can find the books in many libraries and in some bookstores. Some online booksellers, such as Amazon (www.amazon.com) and Large Print Books (www.largeprintbooks.com), carry a wide variety of large print titles.

If you have a medical condition that restricts your diet, nutrition becomes even more important. Take the time and effort to find foods that you enjoy. Consult a specialty cookbook, available for diabetic, cardiac, renal, and gluten-free diets. In fact, no matter what dietary restrictions you have, there is probably at least one cookbook that will work for you, and some come in large print editions.

Cook large batches

To reduce the amount of time you need to spend cooking, make multiple portions of favorite meals and freeze individual servings for quick, handy meals that you can heat in the microwave oven.

———————————— **MY STORY** ————————————

Packaging Takeout and Homemade Food for the Freezer

I have food restrictions imposed by a medical condition. In 2005, after six months of steady weight loss, my doctor diagnosed celiac disease, which is an intolerance to gluten. The treatment is to eat no wheat, oats, rye, or barley. Although gluten-free foods are becoming more commonly available, I wasn't satisfied with the frozen dinners I found. Then I discovered that many Indian and Thai foods were gluten free, and I found excellent local restaurants specializing in these cuisines.

Now I purchase, for takeout, a selection of entrées from these restaurants and freeze them for quick meals that are ready after four minutes in the microwave oven. Before freezing, I divide each entrée into two or three portions, as the servings are so large. I also make large batches of home-cooked food such as chili, and freeze the leftovers.

Round, square, or rectangular? I use different shapes of microwavable plastic storage containers for different items, based on the main ingredient. I store chicken dishes in round containers, beef dishes in rectangular containers, and chili in square containers.

I place each container shape in a different section of the freezer shelf—left, middle, and right. When I decide which

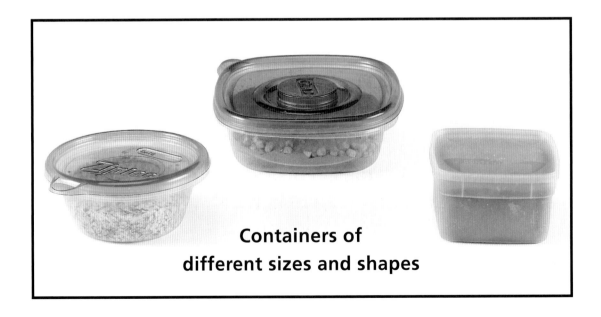

Containers of
different sizes and shapes

one I want, I can pull it out of the freezer almost without looking. Then I place the container in the microwave oven, close the oven door, and push the one-minute button four times. Once the food is heated, I dump the food into a bowl so I don't have to worry about spills, and I enjoy a meal that has been no work to prepare and that is tastier and often cheaper than any frozen dinner I could buy in a store.

Using identification techniques when eating

These tips make it easier to find the food you are looking for when eating, making mealtime more enjoyable.

- Use color contrast to help locate items at your place setting. Put dark dishes on white placemats, and light dishes on dark placemats.

- Use colored or patterned drinking glasses rather than transparent glasses so you can see them and avoid knocking them over.

- Avoid plates with patterns, which can be visually confusing when you are trying to locate your food.

- Use tactile markers to help distinguish items such as salt and pepper by putting a rubber band around the pepper to tell it from the unmarked salt.

- Identify foods by exploring your plate with your fork, or ask someone to describe the location of different items—what's at the top, bottom, right, and left on the plate. Or use the clock-face method to describe each food's position—for example, that peas are at three o'clock, meat at six o'clock.

■ Position your plate so that the meat is nearest to you, as this is the easiest position for cutting.

Going out to eat

Eating at a restaurant need not be frustrating. Follow these tips, and enjoy your meal in confidence.

Seating in a restaurant

■ Ask for a table or booth where the lighting is the brightest.

■ If you are troubled by glare, ask to be seated where glare is not present or where blinds can be drawn.

■ If you are hard of hearing, ask for a table where the level of noise is low. See page 55 for more tips on choosing where to sit in a restaurant when you have hearing loss.

Reading menus

■ Bring along a flashlight that's placed in a Flashlite Friend to help you read the menu. See pages 34–35 for information on this handy device.

■ A magnifying glass with a light helps in reading small print.

- If you are unable to read the menu, ask your dining companion to read it out loud for you—this can prompt some fun discussions.

- If you are dining alone and are unable to read the menu, ask the server to read the sections, such as appetizers, main courses, or desserts that interest you.

- You can avoid the menu entirely by asking the server for the specials of the day or for his or her personal recommendations.

- Decide on your selections before you leave home by checking the restaurant's website to look to look at the menu and decide what you are going to order before you leave home.

Eating in low light

- Select finger food or easy-to-eat dishes that don't require a lot of cutting and that are easy to distinguish on a plate.

- Ask that meat be cut in the kitchen.

- Bring out your Flashlite Friend and point its light onto your plate.

- And laugh when you completely miss what you're aiming for with your fork and try to spear the table instead.

Organizing Your Living Space

HAVE YOU ACCUMULATED all sorts of stuff over the years? If you have lived in the same place for a long time, it may be difficult to follow the common advice to sort through all these possessions and keep only what you really want and use. If you have recently downsized to a smaller place, this task won't be as hard as it is for someone like me, who continues to live in the same house since 1965.

In addition to organizing the things where you live, analyze your living quarters to make sure there are no safety hazards, such as obstacles you might not see. You can also maximize the visibility of large objects such as furniture. Some low vision organizations make home visits to check the safety of your home and offer help in making it safer.

Ideas presented in this chapter are good examples of how you can make your life easier by doing things in new ways. You can develop systems that work for you.

Sorting and storing or tossing

For people with declining vision, it is especially important to get started on downsizing and organizing right away, before it becomes more difficult to see what you are dealing with. Another reason for doing the weeding now is that, if you don't do it yourself, someone else will end up doing it later. Is that what you'd want?

Before you get to work on organizing what you have, get rid of anything you don't need. Sort through your closets and drawers and toss or give away things you do not use.

Giving away clothing

If you have "vintage" or valuable clothing that is in good condition, you could take it to a consignment shop, but first ask your children if they want any of these items. In many communities, charitable organizations will pick up clothing (and, sometimes, household items and furniture that you no longer want). The point is to clear out your closets, bureau drawers, and shelves of things you no longer use. This leaves fewer things to search through when looking for what you want to wear.

Looking at mementos

When you go through your possessions, set aside things you think your children or other loved ones would like to have. It would be even better to have one of them help you with this task, because seeing precious things that have been stashed away can be an emotional experience. What may seem a difficult undertaking can be turned into a special time with a child when you share the history of an item that has sentimental meaning.

Organize photos in one place. You might want to go through them with family members and tell them a bit of family history or remember happy occasions together. Write the names of the people in the photo and add the date for future identification. Have your favorite photos enlarged, or scan and print for placement in simple frames for yourself and the people pictured in the photos. Perhaps the most difficult task is to sort through letters and cards you have been keeping. It helps to be in the right mood—this is a sentimental task, and one that may be best done by you alone.

─────────────── **MY STORY** ───────────────

History for My Daughter and My Farewell to "Dating" Dresses

My daughter learned a lot about me when I told her my history with each dress in an old closet in the basement.

I hadn't looked at them in twenty years and dreaded seeing their condition after all that time of improper storage. Without the support of my daughter, I could not have gone through that closet. Actually, she was the one who took the dresses down from the clothes rod, one by one. I was not up to the task because I hated to think how my precious dresses might look. Each elicited a story, mostly about a special date with her father, occasions that remained vivid memories. She was enthralled to hear about the early days of her dad and me, but remembering those happy times was an emotional and nostalgic experience, especially because my husband had died only a few weeks earlier. It was also sad to see that the dresses were now full of holes. My daughter convinced me that there was no point in hanging onto them and that we should take care of matters then and there. I made my sad farewells. My daughter directed me to go take a nap and after I got up, the dresses were gone. She had taken care of their disposal out of my view, for which I was thankful. I learned what for me was a hard lesson—that I don't need the actual object to keep its cherished memory. Realizing this has helped me in sorting through and discarding other items that were once important to me.

Putting everything in its place

As you proceed with the weeding, you can start finding places for everything you are going to keep. If you are having difficulty seeing particular groups of items, think of new places you could put them.

Finding things in drawers

Try to keep clothing you use frequently, such as underwear and socks, in an upper, easily reached drawer of a bureau, where it is less difficult to see what's in the drawer and reach for what you want. It can become almost impossible to see items in a bottom drawer because lighting is poor near the floor and bending over may be difficult. For me, even a flashlight does not help. If there is furniture in your bedroom with high drawers, but a partner with better vision is using them, try to make a trade of a couple of drawers.

Boxes are a help in organizing and finding things in drawers—and many other places. Be on the lookout for boxes that fit inside your drawers. Shoe boxes work well for small items—you can put particular colors of underwear or socks in them. If you find a particular kind of sock you like or an undergarment that fits just right, think about stocking up on that item so you have a supply and won't need to shop later and perhaps find that the product is no longer available.

Arranging shirts and pants in closets

If you're like me and have a plain, old-fashioned closet with clothes rods, but no fancy organizers, these tricks are helpful, and they don't cost anything. Of course, the first step is to get rid of all those clothes you haven't worn recently. Then you can organize the remaining clothing. Here are several ideas. You may start with one method and later need a different way to identify colors. Experiment to find what works best for you over time.

- Use white garments to separate the various colors of tops and shirts. The colors of my clothes are organized in my closet in this way: white, pink, white, black, white, blue, white, brown.

- When certain items go only with each other, hang them side by side.

- Leave the white paper on hangers from the dry cleaners to provide color contrast, making it easier to see what is on the hanger.

- Use colored plastic hangers or padded hangers in various designs. You can hang blue tops on blue hangers, brown on brown—or, for contrast, brown tops on beige hangers and beige tops on brown hangers.

- If none of the above methods works for you, try the "safety pin method." This system can be used for all types of clothing, from shirts and pants to jackets and dresses. Use safety pins to identify colors by fastening a certain number of pins in the back labels or side tabs of each color of clothing. Because black is the most common color, leave black clothes free of safety pins—that can be their code. Here is an example of the system.

Black—no pin
Brown—one pin
Navy—two pins
Green—three pins

- Shoes can be difficult to identify by color, especially if you have the same style in more than one color. You can use the same color coding system, but use clothes pins instead of safety pins. For example, you might clip together a pair of brown shoes with one clothes pin, and a pair of navy shoes with two pins. Or keep the brown pair in its box to distinguish it from the black pair.

Organizing jewelry

If you have lots of earrings, pins, necklaces, or other jewelry, sort out the things you wear frequently and try these ideas for organize them.

Use an inexpensive plastic organizer, available at craft stores, and put different color earrings and other small jewelry pieces in the transparent compartments. For my earrings and small pins, my organizer has fourteen small compartments in two rows. Each row locks separately, and each compartment has a tight lid that won't open until the row is unlocked by pushing a little button on the side. Several pairs of earrings can fit into each compartment.

Another idea is to find small boxes of different colors and place jewelry of the same color in the box, securing with a rubber band.

Try these ideas or find a different system that makes sense to you. Be a creative problem solver in finding systems that make sense to you—not just for jewelry but in all areas of your life.

Place small items in boxes on the bathroom vanity

A great idea—that can be used in every room—is to use boxes to hold small, frequently used items such as dental floss, deodorant, lip balm, night cream, comb, razor, and shaving lotion. Use a box that is large enough to hold the items in one layer so nothing is buried. This avoids the frustration in trying to find things inside the dark medicine cabinet or scattered somewhere around the vanity.

Organizing your medicine cabinet

Start organizing your medicine cabinet by disposing of items you no longer use and medications that have passed their expiration dates. Keep bottles of pills and other medicines and supplements that you take regularly, such as the AREDS formula, in a special place as described on pages 19–20. Over-the-counter medicines that you take occasionally are more handy if kept in your bathroom cabinet. Arrange like products such as lotions, hair and nail care products, and other personal care products together or on separate shelves, if available. Place each item in a special place so you will always be able to find it.

Filling prescriptions

To save a lot of time and trouble in getting refills, ask your doctor to write each prescription for a three-month period, if paying for the larger quantity fits your budget. See if your pharmacy offers large print copies of the bottle labels. Some pharmacies use easy-to-read labels placed on flat bottles.

Cutting pills in half

If you need to cut pills in half, an easy method is to use a scissors placed on the score line. There are also pill cutters with a built-in magnifier available at low vision stores. A plastic lid over the blade keeps the cut pieces from flying about. Still, this is a job you may want someone else to do. Some pharmacists will cut the pills for you.

Did I take my pills?
Using pill organizers

Solve the problem of remembering to take your medications at the correct times each day by using pill organizers. Organizers are available at drugstores and at low vision stores.

- If you take meds only in the morning and evening, it is handy to use two seven-compartment organizers, with slots for each day of the week. Get different-colored organizers for morning and evening.

- If you take meds three or four times a day, an organizer with four rows and twenty-eight compartments allows you to get all your meds for the week in one container.

- There are many different sizes, colors, and configurations of organizers—there's even one with an alarm system if needed.

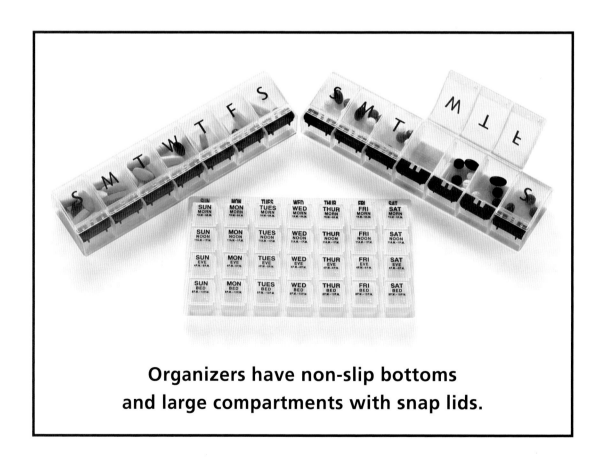

Organizers have non-slip bottoms and large compartments with snap lids.

- Store the bottles of pills that you take regularly in a plastic zip bag so they are handy when you are ready to fill your pill containers.

Avoid bouncing pills when filling a pill organizer

It is easy to drop pills on the floor while transferring them from the bottles to the right compartments in the organizer. Stop the spill by sitting at a table and placing a terry cloth towel under the organizer so that if you drop a pill it does not bounce onto the floor. Begin with all the bottles still in the plastic bag. As you finish putting each bottle's pills in their compartments, close that bottle and place it on the table. When the plastic bag is empty, you'll know you have used all the bottles and you won't have to wonder if you missed a medication. The weekly ritual of filling the pill containers can be a difficult and frustrating task, and at some point you may want to get help.

Organizing your kitchen

You can make things easier to find in your kitchen by organizing your kitchen cupboards, refrigerator, and freezer. Ideas presented here have worked for other people and can help you devise systems that work best for you. Use your imagination to think of ways to adapt the arrangement of your canned goods, other food items, dishes, and glassware.

Identifying and arranging canned goods

Some canned goods are easy to distinguish from others. For instance, it's not difficult to tell a can of soup from a can of tuna. But identifying the kind of soup that's in the can is another matter entirely. Here are some tricks to try.

- Use various numbers of rubber bands: No band for your favorite soup—let's say tomato. One rubber band around chicken noodle soup, and two around vegetable beef. You can use the same system for canned vegetables.

- Use index cards wrapped around cans: write, in large dark letters, the name of each can's contents, and hold in place with a rubber band. This is a handy system because the cards can be used over and over.

- Place magnets with large letters on top of cans.

- If you don't have many varieties of canned goods, you can identify the cans by placing them in assigned locations on the shelf.

Organizing food in the refrigerator and freezer

If you live with other people, designate one shelf in the refrigerator for any special food you may like or need for a special diet. Others in your household can have their own shelves, too. Arrange your items so that each one has a regular place. Use the same system in the freezer—everything in its place. See pages 77–78 for ideas on storing refrigerated or frozen foods in containers. Think about where you place dishes and glasses in your cupboard.

Put the most frequently used items on the lowest, most accessible shelf. For me, this means glasses and cups are on the bottom shelf. The next shelf has dinner and smaller plates of two sizes. The top shelf contains everyday bowls for cereal and soup, along with some heavy glass salad bowls that were a gift from a special friend. Reaching that top shelf is quite a stretch for me. It has been some time since I've been able to see what is in the cupboards when it's no longer daylight, so I use my sense of touch to find or place items on the shelves.

MY STORY

A Broken Bowl Takes Acceptance and Patience—and Not Just For Me

One dark evening I remembered I still needed to empty the dishwasher. I wanted to finish the job before my son came back to pick up his dog after he did some errands. The artificial lighting did not reach inside the cupboard, but that had not been a problem because I knew the place for each item. I reached to the top shelf with one of the good salad bowls, but didn't realize the stack was tipping. The bowl crashed off the shelf, smashing into hundreds of small pieces that landed on the counter and, mostly, the floor.

I didn't want my son to know about my accident, so I started to pick up the pieces myself—a difficult task when I couldn't see them. I got out the broom and swept up some pieces, but I knew others had landed on the rug way over in front of the sink. It was too much for me to handle so I knew I'd have to ask my son to shake it outside—and to pick up the glass shards I was sure I'd missed on the counter and the floor.

I was frustrated and angry with myself for being so stupid. When my son finally arrived, he could tell by my stricken face that something was wrong. When I told him what had happened, Instead of being annoyed, he just started the cleanup. He found large pieces of glass on the counter and I was incredulous that I hadn't seen them. My son expressed no hint of aggravation as he made sure he had picked up each piece of glass. This experience really brought home the fact that it is not just the person with vision loss who needs the gift of patience.

Doing laundry

People with diminished vision face two big problems when it comes to doing laundry—getting the right amount of detergent into the washer and matching up socks from the dryer. Use the following ideas with these tasks.

Measuring detergent

Here are two ways to get the correct amount of detergent into your laundry load.

- As you pour liquid detergent, place the index finger of the hand holding the cap inside the cap to the level you want. Stop pouring the detergent when you feel the liquid on the tip of your finger.

- For either liquid or powder detergent, use a measuring cup or a scoop in the size needed for a particular load.

Matching socks

Even people with good vision can find it difficult to pair up socks as they come out of the dryer. Here are two tricks to make this a snap.

- One way to eliminate the problem is to have all identical socks—one style, one color—so that no matching is needed. Once you find a style you like, buy multiple pairs, and you will not have to worry about matching up socks again.

- If you have a variety of socks, use large safety pins to fasten pairs together at the heel as you take off the socks at night. Color code the socks by using two or more pins for colors other than black or white. If you do laundry for others, be sure that they follow this system as well.

Have a spot-finder buddy

If you live with someone, make an agreement that he or she will always tell you when you have a spot on your clothing or face—toothpaste around your mouth, lipstick on your teeth, or shaving cream under your ear. This will be a great service to you, as spots can be almost impossible to see. A buddy system with a housemate or friend can prevent you from going around with embarrassing spots.

Finding and removing spots from clothing

When you find out about a spot on your clothing, try to wash it out right away. If that doesn't work, as an extra precaution, mark the spot with a safety pin and pre-treat that area before you place the garment in the washer. For items that must be dry cleaned, the pins identify the areas that require special treatment.

Ironing

The best way to avoid ironing is to wear wrinkle-free clothes. But if you do need to iron, follow these safety precautions.

- Use a paint pen to place high marks on the iron settings.
- Place the ironing board next to a heatproof kitchen counter.

- Put the iron on the counter, not on the ironing board, while you prepare to iron or need to set the iron down to rearrange an item.

- Pour water into the iron through a funnel.

- Never grope around trying to find a hot iron. Instead, lightly run your hand along the cord to find it. As your hand gets close to the iron, you should be able to feel its heat. Stop before you accidentally touch the hot face of the iron.

- Use your hands to determine where wrinkles are.

Safe passage through your space

Good balance is needed even when walking in your own home, where most accidents occur. See pages 43–44 for ideas on how to improve your balance. Don't trip and fall in your own living space. Identify hazards that could block your way, and move furniture to clear any narrow passageways. If there is a vision loss resource center in your community, call to see if it offers a home evaluation that will spot possible obstacles and hazards and help you find a safer way to arrange your furniture. Loose rugs pose a danger for tripping when they can't be seen, especially if you've developed a shuffling walk and may hit the rug with your toe, resulting in a fall. The safest policy is to remove area rugs.

Climbing stairs

Follow these guidelines when walking up or down stairs.

- Always use the handrail, but consider it a support only—not an indication that you are at the last step. Some rails end before you get to the bottom.

- Know the number of steps in the stairs you use every day, and count as you go up and down so you know where you are.

- If you have a weak leg, lead with the "bad" leg when going down and the "good" leg when going up. Bring your second leg to the same step once the first is firmly in place. For the next step, lead with the same leg you used before—do not alternate legs. You can remember this rule by thinking of the "bad" leg as "going down to hell" and the "good" leg as "going up to heaven."

Bathtub and shower safety

Most home accidents occur in the bathroom. Bathing and using the toilet require good strength and balance. Features that can help to keep you safe include:

- Grab bars near the toilet and in the bathtub and shower
- Transfer bench or shower chair
- Nonskid bathtub and shower mats
- Commode or raised toilet seat

Use a shower bench or chair if you can step into the shower but feel unsteady standing up. A transfer bench is used by people who cannot safely step into the tub. The legs of the bench are on the outside of tub. Start by sitting on the part of the seat that is outside the tub, and then scoot across the seat until inside the tub. There are suction cups on the inside legs to prevent the bench from slipping. With the addition of a handheld showerhead, it is not necessary to stand up in the shower.

A lightweight shower bench fits inside the tub or shower stall; note the grab bar and non-skid mat.

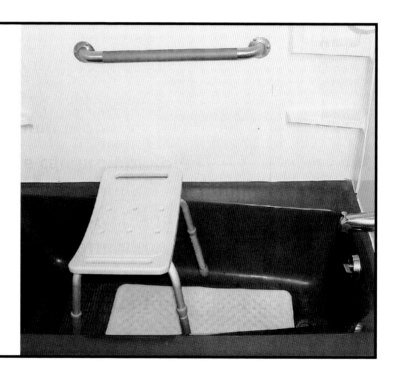

It may be difficult to sit down and get up from the toilet, especially if one's leg muscles are weak. There are no arms, as there are on a chair, to push against to help you arise. A commode with arms is the answer. In the style shown

Transfer bench has legs outside the tub—you scoot across.

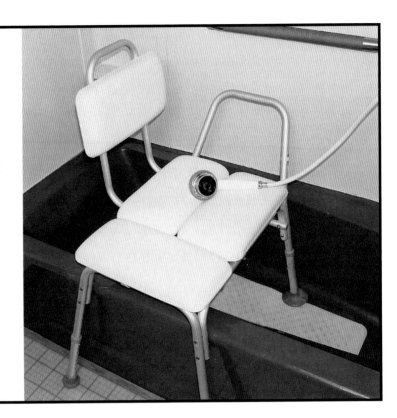

A commode, with arms, that fits over the toilet

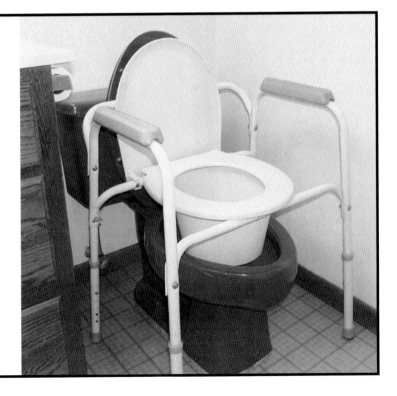

in the photo, no installation is required, and its height is adjustable in one-inch increments.

These benches and commodes are available from medical equipment and supply stores. If it is a medical necessity that you use these products, the cost may be covered by health insurance, depending on your plan.

A bathroom door that swings out of, rather than into, the bathroom provides more space in the bathroom, and the door won't be blocked if someone slips or falls in the bathroom.

Using the telephone

Avoid the dangers of rushing to answer the phone, by placing phones in convenient locations. Ideally, have a phone in every room, and this is possible with a cordless system that comes with multiple handsets, which only require one of the phones in a set to be connected to a phone jack.

Sometimes the only way to have a phone in a handy place is to run a phone line along the floor. If this absolutely cannot be avoided, cover the line with heavy shipping tape or duct tape so you do not trip on the loose cord.

A cell phone is another possibility, especially if you can keep it with you at all times—and remember to keep it charged. See pages 110–111 for information on a large print cell phone.

Battling public doorways

Unfamiliar public doorways can cause frustration. Here are some tips for dealing with them.

- In public places, fire codes require that all doors open to the outside so that people inside a burning building can escape by pushing the door to go outside. This means that you must always PULL the door to enter a public building and PUSH the door to go out.

- Note that a regular door is required to be placed next to a revolving door.

Finding Hard-to-Spot Things

DO THINGS VANISH after you have set them down somewhere? Is the control button on an appliance impossible to locate? Are you not able to plug in an appliance because you can't see the holes in the receptacle or you can't make the plug fit into the holes?

These are all stressful situations that happen throughout the day. If you feel like screaming or crying, or maybe laughing, go ahead—it might make you feel less frustrated. When you've let off the steam, realize that you can still do these everyday tasks, but that you will do them in different ways that will probably take a little longer. Again, your gifts of acceptance and patience—and your sense of touch—can come to your rescue.

Using tactile bumps and marks to identify objects

Small, raised, plastic "bumps" are among the most useful things in my everyday life. Available at low vision stores, these bumps adhere to most surfaces, and they make it possible to find all sorts of things by touch.

Two types of bumps are available. The first are round or square raised bumps that are flat on the bottom that is coated with a strong adhesive. They come in a variety of sizes, colors, and materials. In addition, there are flat

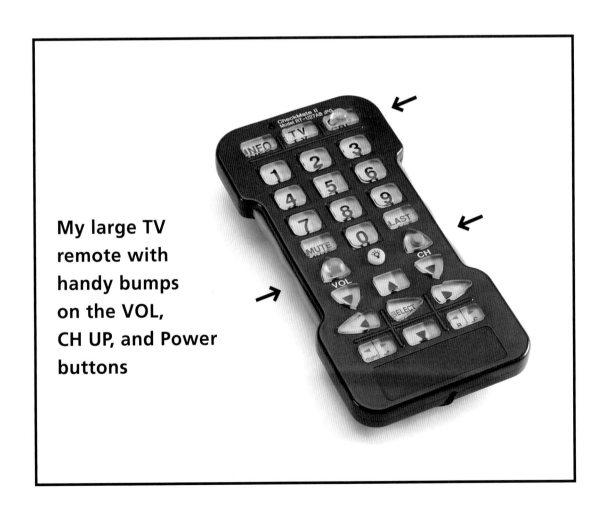

My large TV remote with handy bumps on the VOL, CH UP, and Power buttons

stick-ons made of felt, velour, and cork. They come in darker colors than the plastic bumps and provide different textures to the touch. By using a variety of sizes, colors, and textures, you can distinguish things such as different buttons on a remote control or special keys on a computer keyboard. For example, I've marked the "delete" key of my computer keyboard with a round clear bump, and the "Enter" key is marked with a flat brown stick-on. The cost of the bumps is minimal. They come in packs of ten to forty, depending on the size and material of the bump.

The other type of mark bump is a raised dot made with a pen on surfaces where permanent dots are needed or where adhesive dots do not stick. These raised dots are useful on such items as metal measuring cups and stove dials. See pages 65–67 for a description of how to apply them.

As the years have gone by, I've added the adhesive-backed plastic bumps to more and more items. In my kitchen, I use them on the dishwasher's power button and on the microwave oven's "one minute" and power level buttons. On the TV remote control I have bumps on the power, volume, and "channel up" buttons. Meanwhile, I've used the paint pens to create high marks on my VCR remote control and to draw raised lines on my coffee carafe at the levels I frequently use.

Bumps and high marks can be placed on any number of items—telephone buttons, computer power switches, radio faceplates to mark dial positions of favorite stations, telephones, calculator buttons, keys, dishwashers, clothes washers, remote controls, and other items you want to recognize by touch. Analyze your own needs; then get busy marking items you want to be able to see more easily.

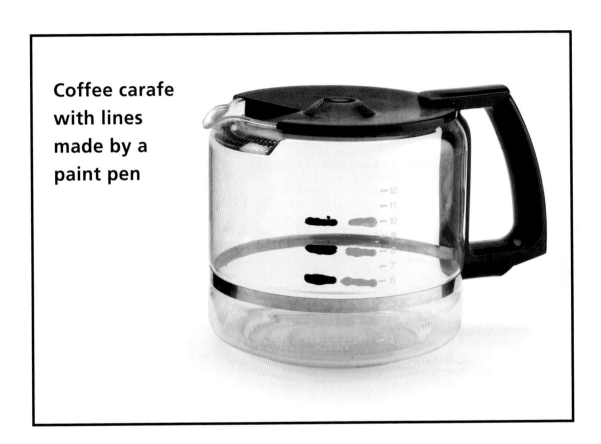

Coffee carafe with lines made by a paint pen

Using white reflective tape for contrast on dark objects

Shiny white tape can make it easier to spot items such as a cordless phone, a hearing aid case, and glasses cases. The photo shows the case for my distance-glasses at left, and the case for my reading glasses at right. I can tell them apart because the tape on the distance-glasses case is at an angle. I use black cases for maximum contrast against the white tape. At the bottom of the photo is a hearing aid case that has been taped with two narrow strips so it can be easily spotted when sitting on a counter.

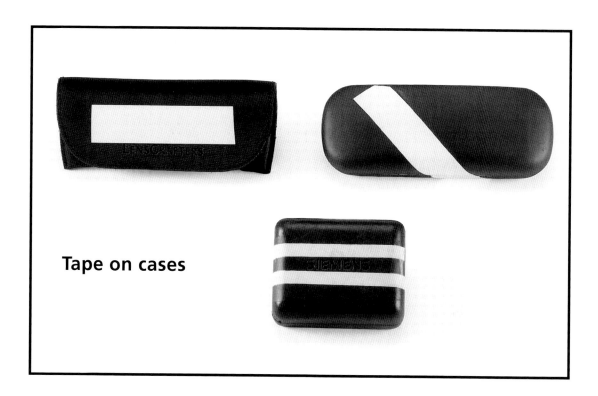

Tape on cases

Choosing a purse, briefcase, or backpack

Trying to find something in a purse, briefcase, or backpack can be like looking into a deep, black hole. Avoid a carryall that is one big pocket, and instead get one that has two or three main compartments and some little pockets in at least one of the compartments. Then figure out what goes in each section, and stick to your plan. I have a purse with side-by-side pockets in the largest compartment—one for my cell phone and one for my tiny wallet, which is about two inches by three inches. I've placed reflective tape around the tops of each pocket so I can see where they are. There are other little pockets for pens, cards, and other small items, too. I always put keys in the small outside compartment. My flashlight goes in the medium compartment along with tissues and shopping lists. My hearing aid case goes in the small outside pocket.

Trouble seeing your cell phone? Try one with large numbers

As more and more features are added to cell phones, the phones themselves have become smaller in size and more difficult to use. Some models are so thin that it is difficult to even spot the tiny phone in a purse or on a counter.

Yet cell phones are useful to people with low vision—for use in emergency situations and to bring along when you are out. Some people no longer have a landline phone and rely entirely on cell phones. But what good are they if you can't read the numbers on the keypad or see the display?

A special phone with a large numbers and a big screen is the answer. The first phone of this sort is a brand called the Jitterbug. Many of the features on this phone are the ones to watch for as more phones designed for those with low vision are available. Here are some examples.

- Large, backlit, bright, easy-to-see buttons on full keypad
- Large text on screen
- Phone list stored on phone with easy access
- Powerful speaker that delivers clear sound
- Caller ID and speakerphone enabled
- Access to all options with simple "YES" or "NO" questions

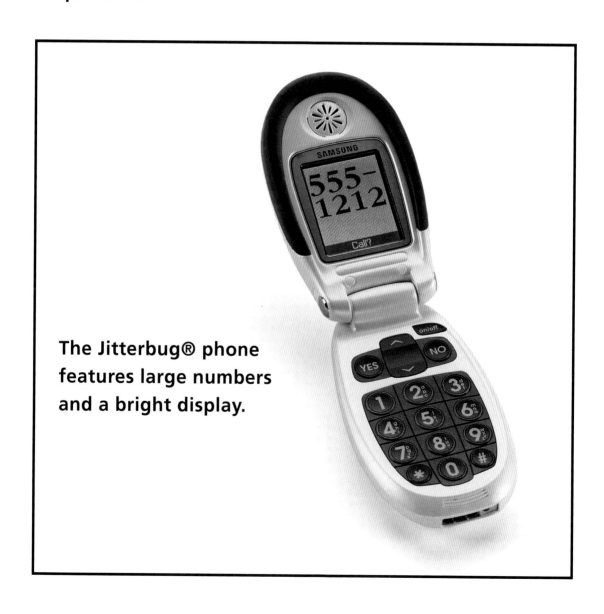

The Jitterbug® phone features large numbers and a bright display.

- Dial "0" anytime feature to reach a friendly operator who will look up and dial a number for you and also add numbers

- Simple text messaging available

- Flip-top design that is large enough to find in a purse or backpack

- Light feature that is activated when the phone is charging, making it easy to spot

- Hearing-aid compatibility, with padded earpiece that also reduces outside noise

- Regular dial tone

Writing with a bold pen— and finding it later

Reading one's own writing becomes more and more difficult as sight diminishes. At first it is easy to read what you write with a pencil, but eventually you can make out only writing done in ink. Then even writing done in black ink can be tough to read. Felt-tip pens provide a darker line and are readily available in many types of stores. If you require an even darker, bolder line, the answer is a Sanford 20/20® pen or a Sharpie Retractable Bold Pen. The pens are available at low vision stores. The ink just flows out of these pens, and the writing is dark and easy to read.

To help spot the pen in a jar, box with other pens, or desk or countertop, I wrap a heavy rubber band around the top of the pen to help identify it. I often find my pen by feel rather than sight—the rubber band works both ways. If it is difficult to read because your lines are not straight, use paper with wide lines one inch apart. I print these from my computer on a form I made.

Getting large-faced or talking clocks and watches

If you are not able to see the time on your clock or watch, you can use clocks and watches with large faces, or get a talking clock or watch—all available from low vision stores. Back in the 1980s talking cube clocks were an innovation. Similar clocks are made today, along with many other styles, including talking clock radios.

———— MY STORY ————

Grumpy is Still Talking

My mother had an early cube clock, shown in the photo. She nicknamed it "Grumpy" because of its gruff male voice. When my children were small, they loved pushing the button on the front of the clock to hear the time. When I recently decided I needed a talking clock, I put new batteries in the old clock and pushed the button. After having been idle for nineteen years, Grumpy loudly announced the time in that same old gruff voice.

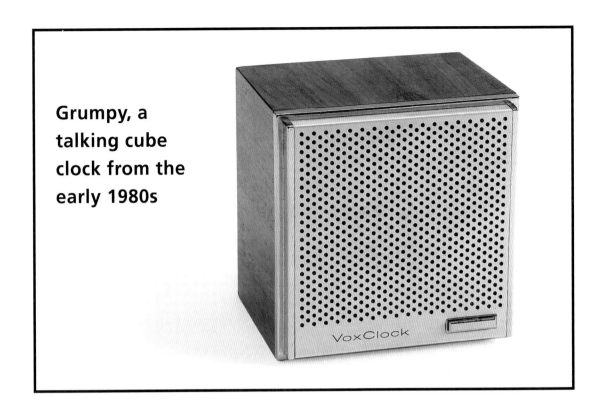

Grumpy, a talking cube clock from the early 1980s

Making furniture, steps, and light switches visible

Here are some ideas on how to make common household items easier to navigate.

- Arrange furniture to provide for an easy route around the room.

- Put white doilies on the arms and backs of dark-colored chairs.

- Put contrasting throw pillows on the sofa.

- Cover coffee tables and side tables with bright fabric or something white—whatever contrasts with the flooring color.

- Place a bright tablecloth or centerpiece on the dining room or kitchen table.

- Use night-lights in hallways, bathrooms, and other rooms you may go into during the night.

- Have a beacon by your bed, such as a radio with a dim light—or whatever light it takes to be able to find your way back to bed if you get up during the night. Keep a flashlight, housed in a Flashlite Friend, on your night table.

- Mark the first and last steps of your stairs with safety tape or tread strips to make them easier to see.

- Use light switch faceplates in colors that contrast with the colors of the walls.

- Put contrasting-colored knobs on cupboard doors and dresser drawers.

- Have a readily available light at the entrance to each room. If there is no light switch by the door, consider adding a lamp that you can turn on by clapping your hands.

Plugging cords into receptacles

To avoid having to bend over or even crawl around the floor trying to find receptacles, get power surge strips with cords that are long enough to allow you to place the strips in convenient places, such as on a side table.

Follow these tips for plugging items into power surge strips.

- Find the wide prong of each plug. Mark that side of the plug with a high mark from a paint pen.

- Find the top end of the power strip—the end nearest the cord that plugs into the receptacle. Position the strip flat on the table, with the top end facing away from you.

- Feel the receptacle to find the side on which the holes with the wide slots are located. Mark the wide side with high marks.

- Using your non-dominant hand, find the receptacle holes. To hold the place, put the pad of your index finger on one side and the pad of your middle finger on the other.

- Using your dominant hand, insert the plug at the end of the cord into the power strip's receptacle.

Finding a keyhole and inserting the key

This is such a foolproof method that it works even when it's dark and you don't know where the lock is on the door.

- Find the key you want on the key ring. Hold it upright in your dominant hand. If there are ridges on only one side of the key, the flat part of the key is the bottom. If the key has ridges on both sides, it may be a bit tricky to figure out which way the key should be turned to go into the lock. You can add a dot on the top side with a paint pen.

- Slide your hand around the door to find the lock.

- Using your finger, find the hole for the key and insert your thumbnail into it.

- Place the key next to your thumbnail.

- Remove your thumbnail from the lock as you slide in the key.

- Turn the key and the doorknob, and open the door.

PART 3

Arranging Your Affairs and Using Assistive Technology

FINANCIAL AND LEGAL aspects of your life are covered in Chapter 8 of this section. Though it is easy to push aside tasks involved in taking care of these personal affairs, they are an important part of your strategies in preparing for the future. Chapter 9 describes ways to enrich and expand that future with the use of adaptive products in audio, video, and computer categories.

Dealing with Financial, Personal, and Legal Affairs

HELPFUL WAYS TO DEAL with the challenges of managing day-to-day finances are available. Simple aids, credit cards, and banking services help reduce the huge frustration that can come when we try to do things that were once so routine, such as writing a check, keeping a check register, and identifying money. Careful planning for managing longer-term legal and financial affairs, including preparation of legal documents—a will or trust, a healthcare directive, and a power of attorney—ensures that your wishes are known and carried out.

Paying bills automatically

Recurring monthly bills, such as gas, electric, telephone, and mortgage can be paid via automatic deductions from your checking account. You may choose the date to have them paid to be a few days after your Social Security and other regular deposits, such as a pension, are available in your account. You can still receive printed statements (marked DO NOT PAY) from the various companies for these bills in the mail or as email attachments.

Writing checks

When it took me an hour one evening to write only three checks and then try to enter them in the check register, I decided it was time to get large print checks. Mine are

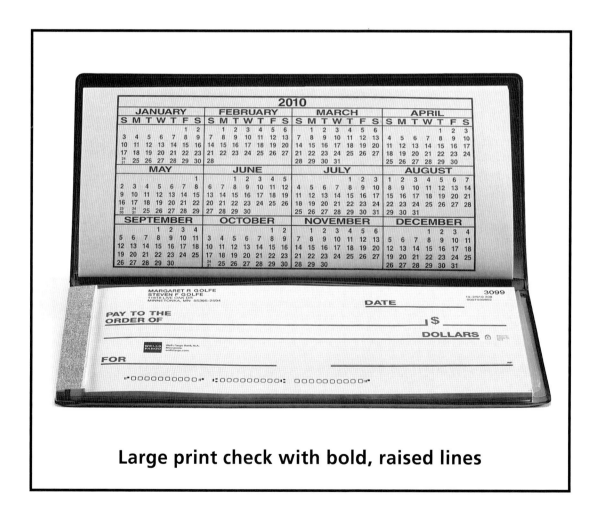

Large print check with bold, raised lines

about 8 inches across and 3¾ inches high. They were available at my bank, and I was not charged for them. They have bold black raised lines, and the background is yellow to help reduce glare and provide contrast. See photo of a large print check.

Another option is to have someone else fill out regular checks, and then you sign them. If you have difficulty getting your signature to fit on the line, you can arrange with your bank to change your signature to just your first initial and last name. Another option is a check-writing guide, which is a template that is placed over a blank check. You write in the cutout slots that fit over the lines on the check. The guides are available at low vision stores.

You can avoid writing and signing checks entirely by doing what my mother and I did when she no longer could see well enough to write checks. She had me added to her checking account, and I handled all her bill paying from that point on.

Keeping and balancing your check register

Fitting dollar amounts in the columns on the regular check registers provided by the bank is even more difficult than writing the check. You can make your own register by using a notebook with lined paper and drawing columns for check number, date, payee, check amount, deposit amount, and balance. You can also custom design a form on your computer and even track the balance on the document.

If you use large print checks from the bank, the check register provided is the same large size with wide spaces for entering the check data. Mine includes monthly calendars. Another solution is to buy a large print check register from a low vision store. The spaces are big enough to write in using a bold pen. Big-number and talking calculators are available to help you balance your check register.

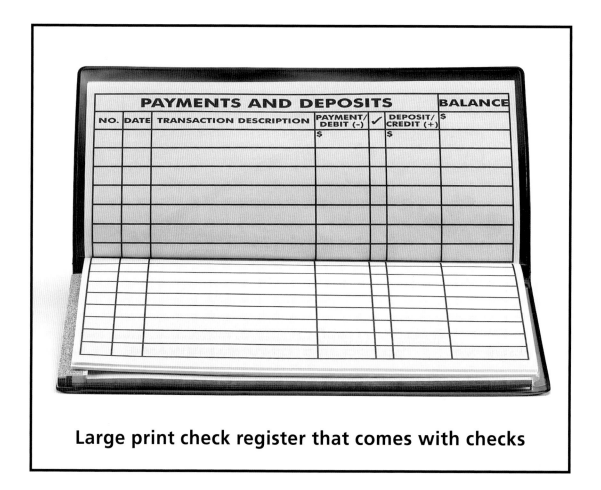

Large print check register that comes with checks

Using debit and credit cards

You can cut down on the number of checks you need to write by using either a bank debit card (sometimes called a check card) or a traditional credit card. With each type of card you receive a monthly statement that itemizes the date and place of each purchase. This listing is handy for record keeping.

When using a debit card, the amount of your purchase is immediately deducted from your bank account. This offers convenience in that you do not have to write a check each month to cover your purchases as you do with a credit card. However, you will be charged an overdraft fee for purchases made when you do not have sufficient funds in your account. Overdraft charges are an unnecessary expense and add up quickly, so keep a record of the amount of each purchase in a register and don't use the card if you do not have enough money in the account to cover your purchase. Insufficient bank funds may also result in a purchase being denied—this is not only embarrassing, but also an annoyance if you have to leave the store without the items you wanted to buy.

Before using a debit card, make sure you understand all the conditions of use. Have someone read you the terms or check with the issuer of the card if you have questions about the terms. Unlike issuers of credit cards, most banks do not protect you if your debit card is stolen and someone uses it to make purchases or get cash at an ATM machine. All the funds in your bank account could be wiped out, so guard your card carefully.

With a traditional credit card, you are sent a statement each month, and if you do not pay the balance in full you are charged an interest fee. To avoid additional debt from high interest rates, consider what you are able to afford and, if possible, do not charge more than you can pay off each month. If you use the credit card for all your purchases, you need to write only one check each month.

If you are a computer user, you can view a history of your transactions online, pay bills, transfer money between accounts, order checks, and perform just about any banking function while sitting in your chair at home.

Identifying money

Finding the correct amount of money in your wallet or coin purse is another new skill that involves the sense of touch. My Uncle Matt showed me a system of keeping track of paper currency fifty years ago. It fascinated me then, and it is still in use today. He folded each denomination of paper money in a different way.

- One dollar: Unfolded
- Five dollars: Folded in half crosswise
- Ten dollars: Folded in quarters
- Twenty dollars: Folded in half lengthwise

If you don't like his system, develop your own or use one of these ideas.

- Put each denomination in a different pocket in your purse.
- Secure five-dollar bills with a small paper clip and ten-dollar bills with a large paper clip. Use no clips for one-dollar bills.

Coins can be identified by paying attention to their sizes and feel. Tell the difference between a quarter and a dime or penny by the coins' sizes is easy, but what about distinguishing quarters from nickels, or pennies from dimes? Feel for ridges on the rims of the coins. Quarters and dimes have ridges that you can feel with your fingernail, making them distinguishable from nickels and pennies.

To find coins quickly, use a wallet with four coin slots (available at a low vision store) or you can use little coin purses for different coins—perhaps quarters and pennies in one and nickels and dimes in another.

Writing legal documents

"Lifetime planning" is a good way to look at the job of preparing or updating your will, establishing your healthcare directive (also known by other names, such as living will and healthcare proxy, depending on your state), and naming a power of attorney. Decisions stated in these legal documents ultimately affect your entire family, and it is a gift to them to have your wishes stated in legally executed documents so that there is no question about what you want, especially in regard to healthcare and how your property is to be distributed.

Making these choices is not exactly a pleasant prospect to think about, but such thoughts may have been lurking in the back of your mind. If you have not yet taken any action, consider that by moving forward, you put yourself in control of deciding important issues that arise later. Take charge of your life by putting your wishes in legal documents and designating who you want to handle the job of carrying out those wishes. If possible, use the services of an attorney who understands the complexities of laws about property rights, taxes, wills, probate, and trusts. If the cost of hiring such an attorney is prohibitive, check with your local legal aid society or the United Way. In many areas of the United States, all you have to do is dial 211 to speak to a government human services employee who can assist you in finding such help. You may also find help from your county bar association foundation, as members often volunteer their legal services.

Preparing all your legal documents at the same time is efficient and cost-effective. Because two witnesses are generally required for all the documents, it is convenient to sign them all at one time.

Deciding how to distribute your possessions and writing a will

A will serves two purposes.

- A will allows you to legally state your wishes about how you want your property to be distributed after your death.

- A will designates and gives legal authority to the person or persons you want to carry out the provisions stated within the document.

Your property includes all your monetary assets and personal possessions, including your pets. Whether your possessions are many or few, it is important to prepare a will so that there is no question about whom you want to receive what particular items in your estate. Be very specific. Just telling a daughter or niece that you want her to have the afghan knitted by your mother does not necessarily mean she will get it. Oral promises are not legal documents, so put such gift directions in writing. Sometimes surprising conflicts arise among relatives who all want or hoped to inherit the same item—whether it's the turkey roaster or favorite pie pan or something with more obvious sentimental value. Painful family fights can erupt over who gets a favorite heirloom.

Often wills state that the surviving spouse receives all the property, but you may want to give a memento or monetary gift to a child, grandchild, godchild, or friend. Receiving such a remembrance is special for the recipient, as I learned when my Uncle Ted, who was also my godfather, named me in his will. His son, who served as his executor, sent me a check and photos of me that my uncle had been saving all those years. I was touched beyond words. Your will is the way you can confidently make such gifts.

Naming an executor to handle your estate

An executor, known as a "personal representative" in some states, has the job of administering your estate. This involves locating all of the estate assets, paying its debts, expenses, and taxes, and distributing the remaining assets according to the directives of the will. Be sure to obtain the permission of the person (or persons) you wish to name as executor(s) before designating him, her, or them in your will. And let the executor and family members know the name of your attorney.

When you ask a person to be executor of your estate, you are asking someone you trust to carry out your wishes. Even with small estates, this can be a time-consuming responsibility, and it is possible to make arrangements for compensation. The more clearly your wishes and directives are stated in your legal will, the easier you make the duties of the person you have given the honor of acting as your executor.

Saving time and money by being prepared for meetings

Before you meet with your attorney, decide how you want your possessions distributed. Prepare by organizing information about your assets and liabilities. Provide copies of important documents, such as previous wills, trusts, power of attorney documents, life insurance policies, and employment benefits.

Preparing a healthcare directive

You can express your preferences about the medical treatment you wish to receive at the end of your life by preparing a healthcare directive, also known as an advance healthcare directive, living will, personal directive, advance directive, and other names, depending on your state. With this written legal document, you ensure that:

- Your preferences will be made known, even if you become unable to express them.

- The physicians will know whose direction is to be followed in the event that your family disagrees about your medical treatment.

- Family members won't have to choose your care levels at what is likely one of the most stressful times of their lives.

- You have appointed an agent or agents to make decisions in accordance with your instructions about your medical care.

States have differing regulations for healthcare directives. You can obtain information and forms from your state's department of health, and often from your doctor. An attorney is perhaps the best source of information and forms. Many law firms have developed a simplified legal form, and you can have it executed at the same time that you sign other documents. My healthcare directive is a legal form that was developed by my attorney's firm. I liked its provisions, so I used that form instead of the one offered by my state's department of health.

I appointed my son and my daughter as my agents, and I have discussed my wishes with them. It is good to start developing a spirit of openness with your family if you have not felt comfortable talking about end-of-life issues in the past. Or perhaps you have tried to bring up these topics and your children have changed the subject. I wish I had been more receptive when my own mother wanted to talk about what she called her "demise" and her thoughts on how things would be after that distant event. I found the topic difficult, but I now understand how much she wanted to share her thoughts and wishes and that it could have been helpful to both of us.

Authorizing your power of attorney

The person you appoint as your power of attorney is commonly referred to in legal documents as "Agent" or "Attorney-in-Fact." That person is authorized to take any action on your behalf that is permitted in the document.

The form is a simple one that includes a checklist of powers you want to grant, such as handling real property or acting for you if you become incapacitated or incompetent. I have again designated my son and my daughter as my powers of attorney.

Your goal is to assign a person or persons a power of attorney in all matters, with all organizations, as defined in your document. If possible, have your document drawn up by your lawyer. Fact sheets and sample forms are available on the websites of each state.

Heed two warnings

First, be aware that some institutions, such as banks, may offer to draw up a power of attorney agreement that allows your agent access to your bank funds, and that authorizes your agent to write checks against your accounts. However, such an agreement has no legal bearing on any other institution, such as utility companies, credit card companies, hospitals, the IRS, and other organizations that your agent might need to deal with on your behalf. Without the proper, state-authorized power of attorney in place, your agent may be unable even to obtain the information needed to pay a bill or settle your taxes in a timely manner.

Second, many people do not realize that a power of attorney is void immediately upon the death of the person who has given that power of attorney. At that point, bank accounts and other assets may be frozen until the estate goes through probate. This is a good reason for your agent to have additional access to funds for handling outstanding bills and funeral expenses. There are several ways to arrange this. One is to have your agent signed onto your bank account so that he or she can write checks from the account even after your death. You can also have your credit card company add your agent as a co-user of the card, with equal responsibility for payments owed. My son and I "share" a credit card, in part because he is very kind about doing shopping errands for me, but also so that he will be able to use the card to pay my final expenses. If you would rather not add your executor or power of attorney to your bank accounts or credit cards, you might just provide your executor funds, in the form of cash, ahead of time so that he or she has the money to handle funeral and other expenses.

Keeping your documents safe and accessible

Storing most of the originals of all valuable documents in a safe-deposit box is a good idea, keeping copies in your home. A large vault inside a bank is the most common location for safe-deposit boxes. To rent a box, you and the others you want to have access—your agents—must sign a lease agreement. Two acceptable forms of identification are generally required. It is a time-consuming matter to add or remove someone's name, so allow time if that becomes necessary.

- Understand that, in most cases, your designated power of attorney has access to the box any time up to your death, not just in the event of your illness. However, upon your death that power of attorney is voided, and no one other than those you have previously arranged to have access may get to your box and its contents. Some important documents kept in the box might be needed immediately. For this reason, consider setting up your safe-deposit box account with at least one other person who will have unlimited access to the box (and who will assume responsibility for it after your death).

- You will probably have two keys. Keep one in a safe place and give the other to another signer on the box. Let each other know where you keep the key.

- The keys you receive when you lease your box are the only keys that open the box. If you lose a key, report it to the bank immediately. You will probably incur a charge for this. If both keys are lost you will probably have to pay for a locksmith to open the box and replace the lock.

- Pay your rental fees on time—if you don't, any property in the box might be turned over to your state's unclaimed property office. It is handy to have the fees automatically deducted from your checking account on a monthly or annual basis.

- Do not use the safe-deposit box to store documents you might need when the bank is closed, such as power-of-attorney papers or, possibly, the original of your healthcare directive.

In addition to keeping documents in a safe-deposit box, have copies—and, in some cases, the originals—in your home. Some hospitals do not honor photocopies of healthcare directives, particularly if the hospital staff takes issue with any stipulations made in the directive. Note: most paramedics are trained to look for healthcare directives posted on the refrigerator when they come to a person's home. For these reasons, you may choose to keep the original of your healthcare directive there—in plain view, in a sealed plastic bag, to prevent it from becoming stained or damaged—with copies in your safety deposit box, in the possession of your power of attorney, and with your spouse and children.

Preplanning funerals

Some people like to plan everything ahead—even their own funerals. Others don't even want to think about such an idea. When an old friend since grade school developed heart failure, I helped her plan her funeral, down to the details of selecting the paper for the programs and choosing the music from selections performed by a musician friend at her bedside. My longtime friend and I actually had fun working out all the details, and it gave her great comfort to plan the service. On the other hand, my husband did not want to hear anything about the plans she and I were making and said he thought the whole thing was bizarre.

If you want to preplan your arrangements, note that there are formal ways to do so.

- Many houses of worship can help you plan ahead. I attended a workshop at my church and received a form to note my choices for music and readings. The information is entered in a database.

- Funeral homes have preplanning guides in which you can enter your choices for everything from flowers to type of burial. In addition to preplanning your service, you can prepay for your funeral through the funeral home you select.

Although such decisions are not easy to contemplate, making your wishes known can give you peace of mind and can help your family by removing their burden of having to make decisions under the most adverse conditions.

──────── MY STORY ────────

One Day Too Late for My Husband

When my husband and I last saw our family attorney, who was about to retire, our wills were six years old. He advised us to update them, as they were at that point irrelevant because our children were grown and did not need the named guardians. I just stuck the name of the new attorney he recommended in a file folder. Year after year went by until ten more years passed. The wills were now sixteen years old, and my husband was less and less inclined to discuss such a topic. In our marriage, I handled all the bill paying, taxes, appointments, and legal affairs, so it was up to me to follow through and contact the new attorney. My rationale for procrastinating was that broaching the subject would be too upsetting for my husband.

Then his health began to fail and he started kidney dialysis. He became more and more fearful, and I was more scared than ever to bring up subjects such as wills, health directives, and cemetery plots. I finally got up the courage to tell my husband I wanted to talk to him about our wills. He seemed almost relieved to be having the discussion, and he told me to go ahead and call the attorney to prepare wills that would include the changes we decided to make.

Again I procrastinated. A month passed, and in February my husband was rushed to the emergency room and later released to a nursing home. I still did not call the attorney. In March I made the call and learned we needed entirely new wills, along with healthcare directives and powers of attorney. My husband was growing weaker, so I told him about the attorney's sample healthcare directive and its provisions about care in the event of a coma. He said to go ahead with that document and, although this wasn't covered in the healthcare directive, he told me his wishes regarding resuscitation. I think we both felt a sense of relief for having confronted these issues.

After that the attorney and I worked quickly. My husband and I had almost duplicate documents, but it took some weeks to work out all the details. My husband had decided that he would like to give special gifts of cash to our son and daughter, and these gifts were listed in the will in heartfelt language. We made a date for signing the documents on April 18, and I arranged to have a room for our meeting at the nursing home. But on April 17 he was rushed back to the hospital. I called the attorney to postpone our meeting.

Things did not seem that serious, but two days later my husband had sudden complications and was rushed to intensive care. The family and six doctors and nurses surrounded his bed, and the lead doctor presented three care options. Our family knew exactly what he wanted and immediately told the doctors. They started to thank us, and I couldn't understand why. I took a doctor aside and asked, and he said it was rare for a family to immediately know the patient's wishes and to all agree on carrying them out. Often the doctors are confronted with quarreling family members and care is delayed while they try to reach an agreement. Our knowing what to do was a blessing not only to us, but also to the doctors—and to my husband. He died on April 19. He did not see or have the chance to sign the will and the other documents.

My procrastination meant that we had no cemetery plots. At the workshop I'd heard about something new to me—renting a casket for the visitation and service, followed by cremation and placement of the urn in a mausoleum. On the way to the funeral home to make arrangements, I told my children about this possibility and that I liked the idea. So did they, and as I had no hint of what my husband would want, other than being with me, we decided on the rental casket/cremation plan. Our decision was made in the space of five minutes in a car when we were under extreme and painful stress. It was not a good place or time to decide something so important.

A few weeks after my husband's death my daughter was back in town, so it was time to tell her and my son about their gifts. Although I wasn't legally required to do so because our new wills had not been finalized, I wanted to carry out my husband's wishes, and I was able to fund their gifts from our joint assets. After a nice dinner at home, I told them that their father had left them special gifts, and I read his words from the draft of his will. They were surprised and moved beyond words. My deep regret is that I was unable to show them an executed will with their father's signature at the end.

Embracing Technology

OPEN YOUR MIND to the ways you can use technology to keep you connected to your world. Do not allow yourself to become detached from your everyday life, but rather consider the adaptive digital products described in this chapter to find new ways to maintain your current contacts and interests and develop new ones. In this chapter, three categories of products are described.

- Audio technology enables you to listen to books and magazines that are read aloud.

- Video magnifiers display enlarged images of print and photos on a screen.

- Computers and related technology enable you to connect to the Internet, use email, view photos, and prepare documents.

- Voice features allow you to interact with you computer by speaking and hearing.

Audio technology: listening to Talking Books

The lives of people with vision loss have been enriched over the last seventy-five years by listening to recordings of books and magazines from the Talking Book program of the National Library Service for the Blind and Physically Handicapped (NLS), which is administered by the Library of Congress. The NLS is a free program that loans recorded and braille books and magazines in a number of languages, music scores in braille and in large print, and specially designed playback equipment to U.S. residents and American citizens living abroad. Enrollment is open to those who are unable to read or use standard print materials because of visual or physical impairment. Through a national network of cooperating regional libraries, material is circulated to eligible borrowers in the United States by postage-free mail sent right to your home.

Origins and development of the NLS and its Talking Book program

The history of Talking Books and the NLS illustrates how the latest technology can be applied to continually make things in our lives more and more accessible. The NLS was established by the Pratt-Smoot Act in 1931, which provided funds to establish a national library program to provide books for blind adult readers. The service is administered by the Library of Congress. The slogan of the NLS is "That All May Read." Seventy-five years ago, when the first recordings were made available, the format was the 33⅓ rpm, 12-inch disc, which was played on a special machine.

During the next twenty-five years the machines were improved, with many refinements made to their motors and operating features. By 1963 all books were recorded at 16⅔ rpm. Audiocassette tapes were first used for recording in 1969, and the analog cassette book and cassette book machine technology were the backbone of the system for thirty years. New models of playback machines were developed over the years, and in 1990 the first talking book machine with variable speed control was produced. This analog system became obsolete by the early 2000s, and the move to digital technology began.

For a detailed chronology of the Talking Book program, visit the NLS website (www.loc.gov/nls/about_history.html).

The move to digital technology

In 2008 the Talking Book program started the transition to a digital flash memory system that uses a cartridge with a small playback machine that is much lighter than the cassette player. The move to digital technology is expected to be completed by 2012.

The flash cartridge system offers several advantages over the cassette system.

- Smaller size—about 6 by 9 by 2 inches, compared to the cassette player's 9 by 11 by 3 inches

- Lighter weight—slightly over two pounds, compared to seven pounds for the cassette player

- Improved audio reproduction, with control of speed and tone of speech, which provides better audio quality for listeners

- Larger storage capacity—one cartridge per book compared to multiple cassettes

- No need to turn the cassette over and flip a switch to access the other side

- Less storage space required for collections at network libraries

- Long life of cartridges and the ability to replay a cartridge many times while retaining high-quality audio output

- Relatively simple duplication process for libraries to produce copies on cartridges

- Using the BARD (Braille and Audio Reading Download) website to download books and magazines

The second phase of the move to digital technology was the BARD program that made material available for download from the Internet. Personal cartridges that you have purchased have the capacity to hold multiple books. The free service is for active Talking Book patrons. The BARD website offers over 15,000 books and over forty magazine titles. More books are added weekly. Contact your regional library for application instructions.

Enrolling in the Talking Book program

United States residents and citizens living abroad who meet one of the following criteria are eligible to participate in the Talking Book program.

- Persons whose visual disability, with correction, is certified by a competent authority as preventing the reading of standard printed material

- Persons certified by competent authority as unable to read or unable to use standard printed material as a result of physical limitations

- Persons certified by competent authority as having a reading disability

- A competent authority can be: ophthalmologists, and optometrists, registered nurses, therapists, and hospital staff; social workers, caseworkers, counselors, rehabilitation teachers; or in the absence of any of the above, a professional librarian.

How the program works

Once you are enrolled, you receive a playback machine from the regional center that provides the players. You start receiving the free publication Talking Book Topics, which is published every two months and is available in large print, on audiocassette, and on the NLS website, http://www.loc.gov/nls/. The annotated list in each issue is limited to titles recently added to the national collection, which contains thousands of fiction and nonfiction titles, including classics, biographies, Gothics, mysteries, and how-to and self-help guides. There are special sections for children's and foreign language books. To learn more about the books in the national collection, readers can order catalogs and bibliographies by subject from cooperating libraries. Librarians can check other resources for titles and answer requests about special materials.

To order audio recordings of books and magazines, check with your regional library.

MY STORY

From Reading to Uncle Matt to Downloading Books

When my Uncle Matt lost his central vision over fifty years ago, he was a practicing tax attorney who lived in St. Paul, Minnesota. He took the streetcar, by himself with his white cane, to the neighboring city of Minneapolis to learn braille at what was then called the Minneapolis Society for the Blind, but which now is known as Vision Loss Resources. After class he sometimes took the streetcar to our house in Minneapolis, where he spread out his large braille sheets on the dining room table and proudly demonstrated how he could read. Before long he became a volunteer lawyer at a legal aid society.

Uncle Matt's hobby and great interest was the Civil War, and he missed being able to read new books published on the subject. Back then there were a few Talking Book recordings on 33⅓ rpm records, but the program didn't offer recorded books on relatively specialized topics such as the Civil War. (In 2010, the National Library Service holdings online catalog listed 1,617 entries for the Civil War.) To help fill the Civil War void in my uncle's life, my husband-to-be and I made weekly trips to his house, where we took turns reading aloud the new books my uncle could no longer see.

Thirty years later my mother, then in her late seventies, learned she had macular degeneration after the cataract surgery that she'd expected would restore her vision made no improvement. Always an avid reader, her life began to revolve around Talking Books. I visited her every Wednesday, and my main activity was reading aloud the list of new books available and writing down the order for her selections. I kept a log of these selections in a notebook that I still have. Her cassette playback machine was awkward, the sound was poor, and she had to pass over many books she wanted to hear because she couldn't understand many high-pitched female voices. She found it difficult, while listening to a book, to keep track of the many cassette tapes required for most books. Still, with her life enhanced by her beloved Talking Books, my mother went on to live a life of spirited acceptance until she died at the age of eighty-eight.

Now, twenty years later, I look forward to the day when I can catch up on all the reading I have not been able to fit into my life. But I will not be waiting for a visitor to read to me or struggle with cassettes and their playback machine. Instead I will listen to books on a lightweight cartridge machine or, more likely, download books from the Talking Book Internet site. This is an exciting and comforting prospect for me.

Commercial sources of recorded books

In addition to the NLS books you can borrow for free with delivery to your home, books are available for purchase in various formats.

- **Audiobooks on compact discs for CD players**
Commercially recorded books on compact disc are available for purchase at "brick-and-mortar" bookstores and on a multitude of websites. You listen to these books on a regular CD player. List prices range from $20.00 to $40.00, but they are often sold at discounted prices.

- **Ebooks for digital reading devices**
An ebook is an electronic version of a printed book that is available for download from the Internet and then read on

a special reading device. The devices offer several options that are useful to readers with low vision. One can change the text size, font, or the orientation, and the text reflows to fill the available view area. Another advantage is that these devices can hold a huge number of books. There are several brands and each has its own format. Choose one with a large screen and a non-serif font that is easy for you to read.

■ **Devices that include Internet access**
Besides dedicated book readers, there are tablet computers that allow Internet connections, making a wider variety of material available for download, such as magazines, newspapers. The Internet connection also allows you to visit website and to use email.

Video magnifiers: start by using simple devices

Simplicity is the goal as you use technology to connect to your world. If a simple aid, such as an ordinary magnifying glass described in Chapter 3, provides you the help you need, why complicate your life with advanced products that your current level of vision does not yet require? You may have years before you need any special help. You can gradually start using more complex aids as you need them. The goals are to be open to the assistive technology that is there to help people with varying levels of vision loss and to know the types of products that are available.

Enlarging with video magnifiers (CCTVs)

Video magnifiers are often called closed-circuit televisions (CCTVs) because they use a camera to take a photo of the material to be viewed and show a magnified image of that material on a screen. CCTV technology allows for greater magnification than does a magnifying glass. There is, however, a sharp difference in the cost of a video magnifier and a simple magnifying glass, with low-end video magnifiers costing well over a hundred dollars and high-end magnifiers costing thousands of dollars. Both stationary desktop and portable models are available. Variable levels of magnification are available within each unit, depending on the particular model. Some models show images in color—these are great for looking at photos.

Handheld portable video magnifiers with built-in screens (CCTVs)

Handheld magnifiers are made up of a camera and a built-in screen in the four- to six-inch size range. In product catalogs, these devices are frequently listed in the video magnifier category. The magnifiers are placed over the material to be viewed and the image is displayed on the screen. You can bring these portable magnifiers with you to read print material when you are out and about. They are lightweight and fit easily into pockets and purses. They are useful for:

- Reading price tags on clothing items or food labels at the grocery store.
- Magnifying and illuminating menus at restaurants.

Desktop video magnifiers (CCTVs)

This type of magnifier looks like a computer because it has a monitor that is similar to a computer screen. In product catalogs, desktop video magnifiers are generally called CCTVs, or sometimes reading systems. Your material is placed on a viewing table that you move to position it by sliding the table side to side and up and down under the stationary video camera above the table. A magnified image of the text or photos is displayed on the screen. Screens are available in various sizes, and you can adjust the size of the magnification to meet your visual needs. Desktop magnifiers are useful for:

- Reading documents, books, and newspapers.
- Viewing photos.
- Writing checks.
- Recording deposits and withdrawals in your check register.

Handheld video magnifiers (CCTVs) that plug into TVs or computers

With this type of video magnifier, your own TV or computer monitor displays images, so the cost of a handheld video magnifier is much less than that of a desktop model. The device, sometimes called a mouse magnifier because of the shape of one model, is actually a small handheld camera. To operate it, plug the cord of the device into the USB port of your computer or into your television set. Place the material you want to display on a table or desk, and move the device over the material. The camera scans the material and displays it on the screen in the magnification you have chosen from the options available with your brand and model. Handheld video magnifiers are useful for:

- Reading documents, books, and newspapers.
- Viewing photos.

Reading with scanner readers that convert text to speech

Unlike magnifiers that display images on a screen, scanner readers convert written material into spoken words by using OCR (optical character recognition) technology after a printed document is scanned by a camera. To operate this device, you hold the reader over printed material and push a button to snap a picture of the material. Next,

OCR software converts the scanned image into recognized characters and words. Finally, a synthesizer speaks the recognized text. Scanner readers can:

- Read most printed material, including letters, bills, receipts, ATM slips, business cards, text documents, and office memos.

- Read items such as restaurant menus and airline boarding passes (portable units only).

- Save captured images for future playback or delete them immediately—thousands of printed pages can be stored by adding extra memory, and users can transfer files to their desktops and laptop computers.

Portable multifunction scanner readers/magnifiers

This multifunction category includes a handheld portable reading machine that also has magnification and multimedia access to audio books and music. The device has a camera at the rear of the unit, a 7-inch video screen, and two controls—one for each thumb—to navigate through various functions, including:

- Reading restaurant menus, newspapers, magazines, and product labels.

- Enlarging the image of any item.

- Listening to music or books stored on the device.

Computer technology for writing, reading, speaking, and hearing

If you are not already using a computer, now is the time to start. Computers open up new worlds, from keeping in touch with children and grandchildren by email to accessing the Internet and finding information on any topic. If you are nervous about your ability to successfully navigate in the world of computers and related technology, consider that many people with age-related eye diseases have had their first successful experiences with computers only after their vision loss. There are endless adaptive strategies for using a computer, including software programs that read aloud the text that is displayed on the monitor.

Refresh typing skills

You can update and practice your skills by practicing touch typing and training your fingers to know the location of each key. The hunt-and-peck system may work for you for a while, but you will be better served by learning touch typing. Classes are available in community education programs, senior centers, and other locations. SeniorNet is a useful organization that offers both online and classroom courses in locations throughout the country. See page 209 for more information.

Get a large-letter keyboard or stick-on labels

If you have difficulty seeing the letters on the standard keyboard, you can get stick-on labels with large bold letters to apply to the keys. A more expensive option is a special keyboard with large, bold letters with black

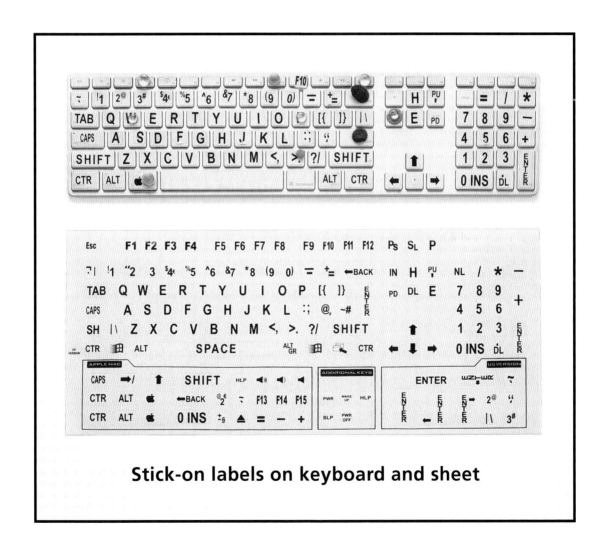

Stick-on labels on keyboard and sheet

letters on white, black letters on yellow, or white letters on black. I started with a black on yellow keyboard; but when I got a new computer and the keyboard was not compatible, I found the stick-on labels even better. I have black on white, but other color combinations are also available.

Selecting a computer and monitor

If you do not already own a computer, check with family members and friends before you purchase one, as someone may have an older model you can use. The more important component is actually the monitor. Look for a model with a screen that can tilt backward because that position may make it easier for you to view text or images. You can change the brightness and contrast levels with buttons on the monitor or through settings on your computer. Experiment until you find a comfortable brightness level.

Using computers' standard accessibility options

Computers come with preinstalled options that help people with low vision see what is on the screen. PC and Macintosh (Mac) computers come with different assistive options; highlights of each system are given below.

Windows operating systems on PC computers

Windows has an Accessibility Wizard that allows you to select different features to help you see what is on the monitor. Here are some of the settings you can change.

- Scroll bar size

- Window border size

- Desktop icon size

- Desktop color and contrast

- Cursor size and blink rate

- Mouse speed

Microsoft Office programs allow you to enlarge the size of the type that appears on the screen. You can also select a font that is easy to read. Tahoma is a sans serif font that comes already installed on most computers. Verdana is another possibility, and it is often used on the Internet. Adobe Reader has a text to speech (TTS) tool, called "Read Out Loud," that can read aloud a single page or an entire PDF document.

Macintosh operating systems on Apple computers

Apple's Macintosh computers contain several technologies to assist you in seeing and hearing what is on the computer screen. These technologies are part of the computer's operating system and do not require special software. Any text can be read aloud within every program except iPhotos. You can also hear a description of what is on your screen. Other useful accessibility features include:

- Zoom options that allow for magnification of up to forty times, with a preview rectangle that outlines the portion of the screen to be magnified.

- Display adjustment options that allow text to appear as white on black.

- Contrast adjustment, for varying degrees of contrast.

- Scalable cursor options that allow you to make the cursor appear larger on the screen so that it is easier to find and follow when you move the mouse.

Speech recognition is available in the Macintosh Leopard operating system, but only for computer commands. You need to purchase a separate software program to have your own spoken words appear on the screen.

Advancing to special accessibility software

There is specific software that goes far beyond the features that come automatically with the operating systems. One category is speech recognition software; another is screen-reading software. The difference between the two applications can be confusing. The distinction is that, with speech recognition software, you do the talking into a microphone and your words appear on the screen as text. With screen-reading software, the computer talks to you through a speech synthesizer and reads aloud what is already on the screen.

Speech recognition software

Speech recognition software is available for both PC and Macintosh computers. After a short training session in which you read a list of words that teaches the software to recognize your voice patterns, you speak into a microphone and your words and sentences appear on the screen. You do not need to see or use the keyboard. For this reason, speech recognition software is especially useful for people with very poor vision and for poor typists.

With speech recognition software you can prepare any kind of document and write email messages. With each new version of software, the accuracy rate increases, but it is a good idea to have what appears on the screen checked for missing letters and incorrect punctuation.

Screen-reading software that requires typing

Screen-reading software is available for PC computers. It works by recognizing and speaking aloud the information displayed on the computer screen using synthesized speech through your computer's sound card. A selection of male and female voices is available to do the reading. Some screen-reading software programs also magnify the computer screen to fit your level of vision. Use this category of software for:

- Creating and editing Microsoft Office documents by typing and using simple commands.

- Hearing a spoken echo of each key or word as you type; you can choose to have all keys or only selected groups of keys "spoken" as they are struck.

- Listening to documents and email read aloud by the speech synthesizer.

- Accessing the Internet and the reading aloud of any web page.

Internet-access software with no typing required

Another category of software enables you to access the Internet and receive and send email without typing. These programs read aloud what is on the screen in the voice you have chosen from a selection of male and female voices. You can also read the screen in a choice of magnifications to fit your visual needs. These require little training and are easy to use.

When you start the program, the software's synthesized voice tells you options you can select, such as email or reading the newspaper on the Internet. You pick which option you want by:

- Clicking the mouse when you hear that option.

- Choosing to have new email messages read to you or displayed on the screen.

- Sending a message by either speaking into a microphone attached to your computer or by typing the message.

The software organizes information in a number of useful ways, including:

- Listing certain sites you can go to directly without navigating the broader Internet.

- Presenting what is available on the Internet in an organized group of broad categories such as news, weather, and entertainment.

- Listing specific groupings within these broad categories—for example, under the news category there are subcategories such as business, finance, and local news by state.

Obtaining technological products

Most of the products described in this chapter are available from one or more of the low vision stores listed in Appendix A. In Appendix C, a list of representative manufacturers and U.S. distributors is presented. By visiting manufacturer websites, getting information over the phone, and visiting stores that sell these items, you can learn about the latest products in the ever-changing field of assistive technology.

The products mentioned in this chapter, unlike those discussed in other chapters, can cost hundreds and even thousands of dollars. If costs are prohibitive, you may be able to get one or more of these products on loan, at a reduced cost, or even free through one of several organizations. Some of these organizations are listed below and are described fully in Appendix B. You need to meet financial and visual-impairment criteria, and you may be put on a waiting list because the products are often in short supply.

Each state has a commissioner for the blind who operates services for the blind and visually handicapped. See page 213 for information on how to find the agency in your state. Agencies usually have products on display, and home visits may be made by counselors to assess your situation and determine whether or not you qualify for state services. Equipment that is given or loaned to you is brought to your home, and you receive instructions on how to use each device.

Lions Clubs in some communities offer assistance. And if you are a veteran, you can consult the Department of Veterans Affairs, which has several programs that offer equipment and training. See Appendix A for contact information.

Forge ahead into the world of technology!

Think of technological products as your assistants in helping you to operate in a world of diminished vision. From the array of product types described in this chapter, explore and adopt the ones that are right for you. Do not be scared off by thinking they are difficult to use. There are people and organizations ready to help you. And if you are not already a computer user, you can give yourself a head start by developing computer skills right now.

PART 4

Maximizing Your Independence

YOUR STRATEGIC PLAN for living well with vision loss includes an important goal—maintaining as much independence as you are safely able to handle. Earlier chapters presented practical ideas for doing everyday things in new ways. This section turns to keeping control over important areas of your life—driving and maximizing independence through the selective assistance of others.

Chapter 10 discusses making decisions about driving. Chapter 11 describes many resources available to help you stay as independent as possible—once you decide you are ready to seek assistance from people and organizations. This can be a difficult adjustment to make. Needing others can make you feel powerless, but consider that it is you who can choose if and when to seek that help.

Making Driving Decisions

DRIVING SAFELY involves many factors, and good vision is only one of them. Strength and agility are also needed because driving involves the use of most of the muscle groups in the body, as explained on pages 45–47. Although loss of the ability to drive safely is one of the most difficult things to face, it can help to remember that even people with excellent vision may be forced to stop driving if they lack the health or motor skills required to safely operate an automobile.

Should I still be driving?

Safety—for you, your passengers, those in other vehicles, bikers, and pedestrians—must be the prime consideration when you decide whether or not it is all right for you to drive. Even if you still have a valid driver's license, you may decide that it is time to stop driving.

Be honest with yourself and you will be the best judge of if, when, and where you should be driving. Ask yourself these questions:

- Do I feel unsafe when I'm driving, even on familiar routes?

- Do vehicles or people seem to appear suddenly out of nowhere?

- Do I have physical issues, such as slow reaction time or inability to turn my head or my upper body, that hinder my ability to check for other vehicles?

- Are other people reluctant to get in the car with me when I'm the driver?

- Have family members or friends suggested that it's time I stop driving?

- Do I become panicky or lose confidence when I find myself in congested or fast-moving traffic?

If your answer to any of these questions is yes, it is time for you to consider whether it is time for you to limit or stop driving. To help you decide, professional assessments are offered by occupational therapists and some rehabilitation centers. Take charge of how to make the decision.

I'm driving for now

If you are still driving, consider adopting self-imposed restrictions such as not driving at night or when it is raining or snowing, staying within a comfortable speed limit, traveling only on local roads with which you are familiar, and canceling trips if the weather is threatening. Giving up driving can be a gradual process with such restrictions.

Renewing your driver's license— the vision test

When the time to renew your driver's license approaches, you may find it helpful to prepare for the vision test by following these tips. Because states vary in their minimum vision requirements for passing the test, cutoff points are not listed here.

- Plan to take the test a few weeks ahead of your birthday—don't wait until the last minute, when you may be more anxious about passing because of the deadline.

- Take the test on a day when both you and your eyes are feeling especially good—a day when you feel confident.

- Get someone to drive you to the test so you don't become nervous just getting to the licensing bureau.

- Ask that your driver come in with you, as you might need help in filling out the renewal application form. When I recently applied, my son had to fill out the form because it was so dark at the writing table that I could not read the questions or write the answers.

Getting a restricted license

If you do not pass the test, you may be eligible for a restricted license if it is offered in your state. Besides wearing eyeglasses, restrictions can include no nighttime driving, no freeway driving, no driving beyond limited areas or routes, and no driving above a certain speed. Some states require a recommendation on restrictions from an eye doctor; others may determine restrictions at the licensing bureau.

Take a driver safety class and get insurance discount

These classes are offered by many different organizations at a reasonable price and are called by various names, including "Senior Driver Improvement Classes" (AAA) and "Driver Safety Program" (AARP), which offers an online course as well as classroom locations such as community centers, senior centers, and churches. At least for the first time, attend a class in person. The give-and-take of class discussions alone is worth making the trip to the classroom.

The basic course is an eight-hour session that is usually offered in two four-hour segments, although sometimes an all-day course is offered on weekends. In most states, insurance rates are discounted for those who have taken such courses. Refresher courses, which generally consist of one four-hour session, can be taken as often as you wish, but to retain insurance discounts, the refresher course is generally required every three years.

In the class, you can expect to learn about current rules of the road, how to operate your vehicle more safely, and how to make some adjustments to common age-related changes in vision, hearing, and reaction time. Here is a list of some of the specific topics that may be covered.

- Maintaining the proper distance from other moving vehicles.

- Changing lanes and making turns at intersections in the safest ways.

- Knowing the effects of medications on driving ability.

- Minimizing the effects of dangerous blind spots.

- Eliminating driver distractions such as eating, smoking, and cell phone use.

- Properly using safety belts, air bags, and antilock brakes.

- Continuing to monitor your own and others' driving skills and capabilities.

Preparing yourself and your car

Before you start off on your drive, prepare for the trip, even if it's a short trip to a familiar place. Use the checklist below to ensure that you are prepared before you get behind the wheel.

- Make sure you have the proper glasses for driving. If you have separate reading and distance glasses, get an extra pair of distance glasses to keep permanently in the car, and store them in a dedicated location.

- Keep a pair of tinted NoIR sunglasses, described on pages 21–22, in a dedicated location in the car.

- Practice this trick for times when the sun is periodically blocked by clouds or when the sun is not bright at the start of a trip and wearing sunglasses would make the road look too dark, but sunny weather is expected during your drive. Keep your sunglasses handy by putting them above your regular glasses or on top of your head, and just slide them down when you're confronted with glare. Push them back up when the sunlight has diminished.

- Assess the weather and check weather forecasts. If rain or snow is falling or is predicted, consider postponing the trip. You do not want to be stranded and unable to drive back home. If it is a sunny day and you are sensitive to glare even when wearing sunglasses, consider postponing your trip or finding another means of transportation.

- Put raised bumps on dashboard buttons, such as those for the heater and defroster, so you can quickly locate them by feel. Practice reaching for the bumps before you drive to see if you are able to find them quickly.

- Check your seat position and mirrors, and make adjustments if necessary.

- Make speedometer readings visible if your dashboard is too dark for you to see the numbers by putting big white dots made with typewriter correction fluid at the numbers for 20, 40, and 60 miles per hour.

- Show fuel levels by putting a white dot at the half-full or quarter-full level.

Driving the car

The following driving pointers can help keep you safe on the road.

- Stay alert at all times.

- Do what you need to do to feel safe.

- Concentrate on the cars ahead, but glance periodically at the side and rear mirrors.

- Know your weak spots, such as slow reaction time or the need for lots of light, and drive accordingly.

- Stay fit and flexible—all parts of the body are involved in driving.

- If you encounter glare from an oncoming car's headlights, avert your eyes and look straight ahead.

- Plan to be home before dark. Check the time of sunset, estimate how long you will be gone, add a half hour for delays, and then work backward to figure out when you must drive home in order to get there before dusk.

"Later" has arrived— giving up the keys

Giving up driving is actually a gradual process. Long before you make the decision not to drive at all, you will probably have had to cancel a trip or find a ride when the weather or other factors prevented you from driving. But the "final" day is one that is long dreaded. Be the one to make the reasonable decision about when that day has arrived. Being responsible preserves your dignity and prevents a "taking away the keys" scene with your children or friends.

Ideas that make it easier to give up the keys.

- Add up the cost of gasoline, car repairs, and automobile insurance for the previous year. That is the amount that you now have to spend on taxicabs each year, with no additional expense to your overall budget.

- Make these savings a special fund. Use a "taxi jar" for ready cash or set up a special checking account where you deposit the amount of your former car insurance or car payments on their old due dates.

- If you sell your car, realize that those proceeds are a one-time windfall. Rather than adding the amount to the taxi jar, consider putting it in a "fun fund" for trips for yourself—not for doctor's appointments or other trips made out of necessity.

- Find a taxi driver you like, ask for his or her card, and call directly when you need a ride.

- Look for a private driver—sometimes a person right in your neighborhood would welcome the opportunity to take you on your trips—and would charge much less that a commercial cab with set rates.

- Ask for rides from relatives and friends, and think of favors to do in return, such as paying for parking, buying a few gallons of gas or a fun gift, or treating them to dinner at a nice restaurant.

Use available door-to-door transit services

In many communities there are low cost transportation services that are available as mandated by the Americans with Disabilities Act of 1990. Besides the low cost, another advantage is that the driver comes to your door and then assists you in getting into and out of the car or van. There may be other passengers. See pages 213–214 for more information. There is usually an application process to become eligible for these services.

Another possibility is to check with Medicaid, if you are in the program, to see if costs of transportation services to get you to medical appointments are covered. If your community has a good public transit system, you have yet another alternative for transportation.

Now relax and enjoy your trips as a passenger. Relish the peace of mind that both you and your loved ones have knowing that you are safe when on the road.

MY STORY

Taxi Al and Other Drivers

Two weeks after passing the vision test for my seventy-seventh birthday driver's license renewal, I noticed a loss of vision in my right eye (that experience is recounted on pages 17–19). I had already become more careful about where to drive, but after learning there was bleeding in my eye and receiving an injection as treatment, I had to reassess my ability to drive at all. A couple of weeks earlier I had called a taxicab company when I needed a ride (to a doctor's appointment) that would have required me to drive on an unfamiliar freeway.

I immediately liked the driver who answered the call, so I asked if he could pick me up after the appointment and if I could arrange rides with him ahead of time. He handed me a card that read, "TAXI-AL at your service." I discovered that he lived close by me and scheduled trips far in advance if I called him directly.

Two days after my eye injection he took me to my volunteer job. I now schedule trips to the doctor and other places with him weeks in advance. We have become good friends, and it is a comfort to have him waiting for me after a difficult medical procedure. He has an arrangement with two other drivers, and if he can't make a trip, he arranges for Clark of Barry to pick me up. Now I have three taxi friends. Then there is my longstanding arrangement with my friend Arlys. We have held season orchestra tickets since 1990, and she became the driver many years ago when I could no longer drive at night. I'm not far out of her way, but it is still a detour. To show my appreciation, I pay for the parking and sometimes treat her to dinner. She is happy with the arrangement, and our bonus is that all those hours spent together in the car have firmly cemented our friendship.

There are other drivers in my life that I can call on occasionally, and one came from an unexpected source. Reiko, my ballet teacher, knew I'd missed a class because of threatening rain—I do not take the chance of being stranded because of a rainstorm—and she asked a young student who lives near me, Amy, to start taking me to and from a summer class, which was held some distance from my home. Because Reiko made this arrangement without consulting me, I was upset and not the least bit gracious—in fact, I called her a mother hen (now we laugh about that). Amy insisted it would be her pleasure to drive me to class and back, but I found that hard to believe. Although it was difficult to admit to myself that I should no longer make that drive, it was even harder to accept unsolicited help. This was a new role for me, and one I am still adjusting to. It has helped that Amy and I enjoy our time together and that we have become fast friends during our trips.

My most important driver is my son. He comes to work in our home office every weekday and, although we have agreed that I will not ask him to use his work time to drive me long distances, he does run short errands for me and he takes me to my regular appointments with my retinologist, whose office is nearby. I do not feel reluctant to ask my children to drive me to important places such as a doctor's office, and I am deeply grateful that they so willingly help me in this way.

Getting Help from People and Organizations

OPEN YOUR HEART and your mind to the prospect of reaping great rewards by accepting help from other people—your friends, family, doctors and other medical specialists—and the professional staff in organizations that are there to assist you. This is another way in which you can use your gift of acceptance.

You can sustain and even expand the horizons of your life by utilizing the myriad opportunities available to people with vision loss. Be proactive and use the information in this chapter to find just the type of assistance you want at any particular time. Calling on others can be a difficult adjustment because it can make you feel powerless, but you are in control of deciding if, when, and where you choose to seek or accept help. Share your feelings with family and friends. Let them know that there will be times when you need to call on them for help, but that you are in charge of your own life and are exploring the resources available in your community, as well as on a national level.

This chapter describes different kinds of help that are available. Appendix A lists national organizations that are particularly suited to people with macular disease.

Not just for the blind

Does it mean you are blind if you decide to use the services of an organization with the word "blind" in its name? No!

The word "blind" is in the names of many local centers, national nonprofit organizations, and government agencies. Do not be turned off or scared away by that word. Some people have been known to refuse to even contact an agency because the word "blind" is in its title. Could this be a rationalization for not getting help?

Note that many longtime nonprofit organizations have changed their names over the years to indicate that they serve people with varying degrees of low vision. Some agencies now include the words "visually handicapped," "vision loss," or "visually impaired" in their names. For example, as mentioned in the MY STORY on pages 146–147, the center in Minneapolis is now named Vision Loss Resources. The Minneapolis Society for the Blind was founded in 1914 and was renamed in 1990 when it merged with another local agency.

Letting family, friends, and strangers know your needs

Your vision loss affects not only you, but your family and friends, too. Realize that they, too, must also develop a spirit of acceptance and patience. They may need to help you with various tasks, but let that help be in ways that are appropriate and useful for you. If you are not the instigator of the idea of such help, you may feel a loss of control. Realize that it is up to you to decide what help you want to accept and when you want to actively seek help in a particular area of your life.

Ideas for handling various "help" situations

Sometimes family and friends do not know how to give you the help you may—or may not—need. It is up to you to let them know what is right for you. Here are examples of some types of people and how to handle situations with them.

- Overly protective people may offer unsolicited help that you do not need. You can be politely assertive and say, "It's important that I stay as independent as possible, so please allow me do whatever I can. I'll ask for assistance when I need it, so don't feel you always need to offer help."

- Those who are oblivious to your situation often ignore the fact that you need assistance in some area—the opposite of being too solicitous. Again it is up to you to let them know what you need. You can say, "I appreciate your thinking I can do everything myself, but I would like your help with (you name it)."

- People attuned to your needs and desires are the ideal helpers, so accept their help with thanks.

- Those who persist in offering help that you could actually use but want to reject because you'd then have to admit that you need it. This has much less to do with other people than it does with you. Ask yourself, "Am I letting pride or denial get in the way of acting in my own best interests?" If the answer is yes, try not to become huffy, as I did (and came to regret) when I didn't want to accept a ride, as told at the end of the MY STORY on pages 176–178.

Asking for—or accepting— too much help

If someone in your life is a very helpful type, it is easy to fall into the trap of accepting or asking for help that you do not really need. Doing so will ultimately reduce your independence. In my own case, I strive to be more aware so I don't automatically use help from my son that I don't actually need. He comes to work every weekday in the home office of our family publishing business.

He is patient and kind and, for instance, if I can't find something right away that I've set down somewhere, I can get frustrated and ask him to find it rather than keep searching for it myself.

Sometimes when I find myself too easily accepting or relying on assistance with some task I could safely accomplish on my own, I remember a gentleman who attended the low vision skills class I took. He had very little vision and his wife drove him to class, but she did not "hang around" during the class to assist him— instead, she went upstairs, did crossword puzzles, and came back in time to join in the lunch we prepared in class. She reminded him that he was in the class to learn to do things for himself. She was reinforcing his need for independence, and she let him know that she was not going to help him when he could do something for himself. This example serves as a good reminder to be conscious of the type of help we are using and to make sure it is at an appropriate level.

Be proactive in communicating your needs

Becoming comfortable talking to your family and friends about your needs may be difficult.

- Be open about telling people how you are feeling so they don't have to try to guess whether or not something is wrong.

- If you are having a bad eye day (or, as one woman puts it, "My eyes are crabby today"), you may need to ask for special attention or help in deciding whether or not you want to participate in a planned activity.

- Feel free to suggest things you really would like from others, such as offers to take you shopping or to a doctor appointment, or fun things like going out to lunch or the opportunity to share gift ideas that you have found in low vision catalogs.

Talking about your vision loss— it's up to you

Sometimes when you are out and about, you may run into situations in which it makes sense to mention you have a vision loss. Remember that, in all cases, it is up to you to decide whether or not you want to say anything. Here are some scenarios and ideas for how you could handle them.

- At a store, you may need help with reading a price tag, or with signing a charge slip at the checkout station when you can't see the line on which to write your signature. Practice a standard line that you can say with confidence, such as, "Please show me where to sign, as I don't see well (or have vision loss, or have poor vision," or my short phrase, "I have bad eyes."

- At social gatherings and other situations, if you are open about your vision, you may have some interesting conversations when the person you are talking with tells you all about a relative or friend with vision loss. I've made some wonderful new connections this way.

- If people become overly inquisitive, remember that you are under no obligation to talk about your vision. You can say, "I prefer not to discuss this," or, "I find it rather boring to discuss my vision loss."

Trying to identify people

Not being able to recognize people because you can't make out their faces or see them can be embarrassing. If someone you know comes up to you at a social function and you can't tell who it is by voice or figure, you can explain that you don't see well. Actually, this may be better than admitting that you have forgotten the person's name, which can happen, too, and is also embarrassing.

You may want to ask even people you know well and see often that they make a habit of identifying themselves when they see you.

Develop a spirit of gratitude for the help you receive

As we continue to make adjustments in our lives to accommodate vision loss we can experience many feelings, but gratitude may not readily come to mind, yet it is an important gift to both you and others. Try to remember to thank the helpers in your life. Let them know you appreciate what they do for you and recognize that your situation makes life difficult for them, too.

Sometimes I think I present a triple whammy to those around me. I have vision loss and need help in many areas. I have a hearing loss—and I don't always wear my hearing aids, so I'm often saying, "What? Can you say that again more clearly?" I also have celiac disease and can't eat a normal diet—no wheat, oats, barley, or rye. My family and friends have immense kindness and patience in the ways they must adapt their lives to fit my needs, yet how often do I remember to let them know how grateful I am for their help?

Using local and regional resources

Besides your immediate circle of family and friends, there are local resources that can offer help and a variety of services in the areas of recreation, transportation, and healthcare. In addition to the special adaptive recreational opportunities described below, assistive services are offered by a wide array of senior centers and community centers, as well as by vision loss agencies that offer a variety of social and recreational activities, which are described later in the chapter.

Adaptive recreational opportunities

Audio descriptions of the visual elements of live theater, selected television shows, and some movies are available to enhance your understanding and enjoyment of these types of entertainment.

- Television. Descriptions by a narrator of visual elements such as actions, settings, scene changes, and body language are provided during natural breaks in the program's dialogue. Check with your local stations or cable companies to see what is available. Also, when buying a new television set, be sure that it can accept audio description.

- Audio-described performance. Theater productions of plays that run for long periods of time (as opposed to those that open and close quickly or that come into town for a day or two) often have performances that include audio descriptions. You wear a headset to hear the narration. Ticket prices are often subsidized for you and a companion. Call your local theater companies to find out if they have these performances.

- Audio-described movies and videos. Visit the following websites to locate movie theaters that show audio-described films by country, state, and city. Call local movie theaters to ask if they show audio-described movies.

- A list of audio-described movies with ratings on the ease or difficulty of following the story is offered by the website Blindspots: Movie Reviews for Visually Impaired People (www.vashti.net/Blind/table.htm).

Talking books and magazines from your regional NLS library

The Talking Book program is discussed more thoroughly in Chapter 9, but these key points are worth mentioning again. You may borrow recorded books, magazines, and playback equipment from a regional library that is in the network of the Talking Book program of the National Library Service for the Blind and Physically Handicapped (NLS).

- The program is available to U.S. residents and U.S. citizens living abroad whose low vision, blindness, or physical handicap makes it difficult to read a standard printed page. The eligibility requirements of the Talking Book program are less stringent than those of the other government agencies listed at the end of this chapter.

- Playback machines for listening to the recordings are provided on free loan.

- The U.S. Postal Service delivers the recordings, which are sent right to your mailbox from your regional library, and you return them, postage free, to the regional library.

- To enroll in the program, you can start the process by calling 1-888-657-7323 and follow the prompts to be connected to the appropriate library. You can also find your library and fill out a request form on the NLS website (www.loc.gov/nls.index.html).

- Your local vision loss agency can help by leading you through the application process and helping you fill out the forms.

Transportation services

Information on transportation services for the disabled is mentioned at the end of Chapter 10. To find transportation services in your area, contact your local Area Agency on Aging by calling 1-800-677-1116.

Medical specialists

Put together a medical team that covers all aspects of your healthcare, starting with your primary care physician, who will take care of your basic health needs and refer you to specialists for specific conditions. Below is a list of some of the specialists who may become part of your personal healthcare team.

- Retinologist. Your retinologist is an essential member of your team. It is important to keep your routine appointments, and it is crucial that you see your retinologist whenever you notice a change in your vision because there may be a benefit from an early treatment.

- Ophthalmologist. You see your ophthalmologist once a year for a general eye checkup and to explore the possibility of improving your vision with a new eyeglass prescription.

- **Ophthalmic plastic surgeon.** If you wish to explore the possibility of surgery to correct drooping eyelids that are blocking your field of vision, this is the specialist to consult. First, get the opinions of your ophthalmologist and retinologist, and request a referral if you want to pursue the idea.

- **Occupational therapist.** To help maximize your independence in your daily activities, an occupational therapist can provide evaluation and training services to help you live with vision loss. See the entry for the American Occupational Therapy Association in the organization list on page 204 for more information.

- **Physical therapist.** Balance and physical fitness are especially important for people with vision loss, and a physical therapist can develop an exercise program to address your particular needs.

- **Podiatrist.** A large number of balance problems originate in the feet, and a podiatrist may suggest orthotic aids to put in your shoes for extra support. A podiatrist can also provide toenail care and remove painful corns and calluses that may be making it difficult to walk.

- **Your own specialists.** Depending on your own health conditions, you may see specialists in various fields, such as an endocrinologist if you have diabetes.

Deciding to seek help from local vision loss organizations

Many communities have a vision loss agency that offers a wealth of services. For some it can be scary to even think about looking for help outside your own circle. You may feel that, by acknowledging your need for more help than friends and family can give, you are surrendering your independence. Just the opposite is true, as you can learn new ways to remain independent and maximize control over your life. Perhaps you feel uncomfortable about the prospect of sharing your story with strangers or about taking a class for the first time in years. But making that first call is a positive step because it shows that you are accepting your condition to the point that you are ready to open the doors to whole new ways of living.

What will happen when I call?

The first step when you call is to set up an appointment for an intake interview. At this interview, basic identification information is gathered, and you may be asked about the history of your disease. In some cases, a staff person also does a simple vision evaluation to get an idea of the equipment and services that might be helpful for you.

What services will I be offered?

A counselor will tell you about the various services offered at the center. Examples from the huge variety of activities that may be offered are listed below, but understand that not all organizations offer all of these services.

- **Computer training**
  Accessibility software for magnifying what is on the screen and for reading aloud what is on the screen, plus software
  Communicating by email
  Keyboard typing skills

- **Cooking**
  Adaptive cooking and kitchen safety techniques
  Recipes in large type
  Special kitchen aids

- **Daily living skills**
  Doing household chores
  Handling money
  Managing finances
  Marking and identifying clothing and other items
  Organizing household items and furniture

- **Fitness and health**
  Guidance in designing a personalized fitness program
  Healthy-eating support groups
  Instruction on using fitness equipment
  Yoga and workout classes
  Walking groups

- **Filling out forms**

  Assistance with filling out forms such as applications for Talking Books or mobility services

  Help with filling out income tax returns

- **In-home evaluation**

  Development of a plan of service

  Identification of needs for magnifiers, lighting, etc.

  Information on other community resources

- **Leisure and recreation**

  Craft classes and groups in such areas as basket weaving, woodworking, soap making, and jewelry making

  Needlework classes and groups in such areas as knitting, crocheting, and quilting

  Bingo, cribbage, and board games

  Book clubs that use books on tape

  Card games such as hearts, bridge, and poker

  Journal and creative writing classes and groups

  Lunch and supper club outings

  Movie showings with audio descriptions

  Trips to museums and plays

- **Library**

  Audio books

  Audio-described videos and DVDs

  Large print periodicals and books

- **Support groups**

  Support and socialization with peers who understand your challenges, meeting in groups moderated by a staff person or a trained volunteer facilitator

- **Volunteers and volunteering**

  Help with shopping, reading, and leisure skills

  One-on-one peer counseling with trained, visually impaired volunteers

  Opportunities to become a volunteer yourself!

- **Miscellaneous**

  Free Bible on tape

  Free directory assistance for your telephone

  Large print or amplified phones, if you also have hearing loss

  Mobility transportation services

  Talking Books, radio, and newspaper reading services

- **Presentations about agency services**

Many low vision agencies provide speakers for people living in various types of residences, such as assisted living or long-term care faculties, and to members of organizations such as senior centers. If you would like to arrange for a speaker for your group, contact your local agency. Many low vision agencies also have speakers who provide information on vision loss to other professionals.

National organizations—programs and services

There are an estimated 1,400 organizations across the United States devoted to helping individuals and their families adapt to living with vision loss. See Appendix B for descriptions of organizations that are especially useful to people with macular disease.

───────────── **MY STORY** ─────────────

Why Did it Take Me So Long?

I keep notes of every visit with my retinologist, and every now and then I remembered making a note about a counselor at Vision Loss Resources, a local vision rehabilitation agency, whom the doctor had mentioned on more than one visit. I had asked if there were any support groups, and the referral was in response to my question. I just kept the idea of calling the counselor pretty well buried in the back of my mind until my retinologist brought it up again during subsequent visits. Still, I did nothing.

When I finally made the call to the counselor, I checked my notes and found that it had been four years since the doctor first told me about her. By then it had been eight years since my initial diagnosis. The benefits of meeting with the counselor have been enormous. Perhaps the most important benefit is that, by taking that first step, I finally had become ready to go after help on my own.

At that first meeting I kept hearing peals of laughter from the next room, and I was invited to join the group of men and women who were having a wonderful time eating the lunch that the cooking instructor had prepared in a demonstration. The people in this group had severe vision loss. I was seated next to two women who were members of the organization's advocacy group and who were involved in community education. They go out to various facilities and tell groups about the services offered by the center. The women also had received training to become paraprofessional aides to assist staff members who moderate support groups. These inspiring women showed me how much someone with severe macular disease could contribute, even when living with only peripheral vision.

Enrolling as a client at the center changed my life. My resolve to keep a positive outlook was affirmed and bolstered by meetings with my counselor, and other staff members have guided me in various ways. I have met inspiring people with vision loss in classes and at various functions at the center. In a weekly life skills class I learned many new ways to live my life, including special cooking techniques, how-to ideas for the all-important organization skills I need, and an upbeat approach to dealing with the frustrations of living with vision loss.

Why did I wait so long to take the first step in seeking help? My counselor told me that it was because I was not ready earlier. She said that people come at all stages of their disease, and that there is not a single "right" time for everyone. The right time is when one is ready. Sometimes I wish I had been ready earlier, but I think a streak of stubbornness got in my way. When others in my class who were at later stages of vision loss had difficulty reading the recipes printed in giant-size type, I kept thinking, "If only they had come sooner, they could have been using these practical ideas for years." Then I remembered that the same wisdom applies to me.

In the introduction to this book, I said
my goal was to offer hope.

I keep hope by remembering that
there will always be one more thing to try.
I live with hope, and you can, too!

Low Vision Stores

ALMOST ALL of the products mentioned in this book are available at one or more of the three low vision stores listed below. There may also be local stores in your community where you can see and buy some of the products. Amazon.com also carries many of the products mentioned in the book.

independent living aids, inc.
PO Box 9022, Hicksville, NY 11802
800-537-2118
www.independentliving.com

LS&S
1808-G Janke Drive, Northbrook, IL 60062
800-468-4789
www.lssproducts.com

Maxi-Aids, Inc.
42 Executive Boulevard, Farmingdale, NY 11735
800-522-6294
www.maxiaids.com

National Information Sources, Programs, and Services

Some national organizations that provide important advocacy, education, and research functions, as well as especially useful services to people with macular disease, are described below. The especially useful services fall into two categories:

- Locators that provide assistance in finding specific services in your community, such as chapters of national organizations, state services, talking radio stations, and many others.

- Publications that feature news of the latest research developments and that list centers for computer training.

Browse the list to find what appeals to your interests; then contact the service to find out what it can do for you.

American Foundation for the Blind (AFB)

800-232-5463

www.afb.org/seniorsite

The AFB's mission is to broaden access to technology, elevate the quality of information and tools for the professionals who serve people with vision loss, promote independent and healthy living for people with vision loss by providing them and their families with relevant and timely resources, and maintain a strong presence in Washington, DC, to ensure that the rights and interests of people with vision loss are represented in public policies.

The AFB Senior Site offers many excellent menu options, including an online directory of more than 1,500 organizations in the United States and Canada that provide services such as computer training, counseling, support groups, and classes in independent living skills. Explore other features on the toolbar, such as "Newsletters," for a list of four free email newsletters.

For assistive products and manufacturers go to www.afb.org and enter "Products" in the search box. For reviews of assistive products, enter "Product evaluations" in the search box.

American Macular Degeneration Foundation (AMDF)

888-622-8527

www.macular.org

Find a state agency: www.macular.org/stagency/index.html

Find a support group: ttp://www.macular.org/sgroups/mnsg.html

Canadian services: http://www.macular.org/canada.html

International services: http://www.macular.org/internat.html

Publication: http://www.macular.org/spotlite.html

The newsletter SPOTLIGHT provides scientific information, including recent research. It is available for a $25.00 annual donation. See http://www.macular.org/spotlite.html

The American Macular Degeneration Foundation works for the prevention, treatment, and cure of macular degeneration by raising funds, educating the public, and supporting scientific research. Services include vocational rehabilitation and job placement services, financial assistance or referrals to other agencies or organizations that provide similar services in the community, orientation and mobility training, and transportation services.

American Occupational Therapy Association, Inc. (AOTA)

301-652-2682

www.aota.org

Find a driving evaluator: http://www.aota.org/
    Older-Driver/Consumer/Evaluate/Eval-by-OT.aspx

The AOTA is an official association of occupational therapists in the United States. Many therapists are trained to conduct driving evaluations. If there is no specialized vision loss agency in your area, these professionals can help you with many of the things you would learn at a specialized agency, including cooking, marking items for easy identification, developing senses besides sight, and using assistive devices. These services are provided in your home, and suggestions could be made about your lighting and furniture arrangements.

Better Health for Better Vision

www.WebRN-MacularDegeneration.com

Newsletter subscription: click Free Newsletter near the
    top of the menu bar.

Newsletter archive: http://www.webrn-
    maculardegeneration.com/WebRNMacular_
    Degeneration_News-backissues.html

The goal of this health-oriented weekly email newsletter and website is to raise awareness and knowledge of macular degeneration. By covering topics such as the causes, symptoms, and treatment of macular degeneration, it works to bring hope to those who have been diagnosed with the disease. There is special emphasis on new assistive products and on medical advances. On the informative website, categories of topics include the risks, causes, and treatment of macular degeneration; research and clinical trials; diet and supplements; and helpful aids such as many types of magnifiers.

Foundation Fighting Blindness (FFB)

800-683-5555
www.blindness.org

The mission of the FFB is to drive research that leads to the prevention, treatment, and cure of retinal disease. The website offers a choice of type sizes and a wealth of information on its pages. More than fifty volunteer-led chapters raise funds, increase public awareness, and provide support to each other and their communities. The VisionWalk program is the national signature fundraising event since its inception in 2006. Walks are sponsored by individual chapters.

FFP has funded thousands of research studies in promising areas such as genetics, gene therapy, retinal cell transplantation, artificial retinal implants, and pharmaceutical and nutritional therapies. The FFB provides information and outreach programs for patients, families, and professionals. The website lists current clinical trials and features pages on retinitis pigmentosa, macular degeneration, Usher syndrome, and a large spectrum of other retinal degenerative diseases. *InFocus*, mailed three times a year to members, reports on research, science news, and FDA-approved clinical trials.

International Association of Audio Information Services (IAAIS)

800-280-5325
http://iaais.org/index.html

The IAAIS is a worldwide volunteer-driven organization of over a hundred independent Audio Information Services that turn text into speech for those who are unable to read or hold printed material. Most services use volunteer readers, and many U.S. stations are associated with public radio stations, colleges and universities, and libraries. The IAAIS website offers a large type option and includes a directory of radio stations that provide immediate, verbatim audio access to newspapers, magazines, consumer information, and selected material such as public affairs programs, books, and daily exercise programs.

Some services also offer a variety of related programs, such as personal reader programs; audio-description services of live theater, museum exhibits, nature trails, parades, and other visual venues; audio transcription; taping services; and other audio-based community services.

Lions Clubs International

630-468-6901

www.lionsclubs.org

Lions Club International has over 45,000 clubs and 1.35 million members, making it the world's largest service club organization. The website, offered in a multitude of languages, includes a Find a Club link. For nearly 100 years, its members have worked to prevent blindness, restore eyesight and improve eye care for hundreds of millions of people worldwide. Local clubs may sponsor programs for the visually impaired and may donate aids such as talking clocks and, sometimes, computers to people who are visually impaired. Some clubs provide large print books to libraries. Lions Club services may include supporting guide dog schools, scholarships for blind students and vocational training programs, facilitating self-help groups, and supporting recreational activities and Lions camps for the blind/visually impaired.

Macular Degeneration Partnership

310-623-4466

www.amd.org

Publication: AMD News Update, an email newsletter, features excellent information regarding current research on both the dry and wet forms of macular degeneration.

The Macular Degeneration Partnership is an outreach program of the nonprofit Discovery Eye Foundation with a mission to provide comprehensive, easily understood, and up-to-the-minute information about macular degeneration to the public through the Internet, telephone, public events, and printed materials. The organization's goal is to support research and coordinate advocacy efforts.

Macular Disease Society (United Kingdom)

01 264 350551
www.maculardisease.org

This British organization is a self-help society for those diagnosed with any of the eye conditions that fall under the classification of macular disease. The society is dedicated to providing information and practical support so that those with the condition may make the most of their remaining vision. The informative website promotes independence, confidence, and quality of life; promotes and funds research into macular degeneration; and hosts a discussion forum for its members, covering many topics.

Prevent Blindness America

800-331-2020
www.preventblindness.org

Founded in 1908, Prevent Blindness America is a volunteer eye health and safety organization whose sole mission is the prevention of blindness and the preservation of sight. The organization offers education programs, screenings for vision problems in adults at locations such as senior centers and for vision problems in children in schools, training and certification for people around the country to conduct screenings, and various community and patient service programs, including an email newsletter. The website lists affiliates in the several states where they are available. Prevent Blindness America advocates at the local, state, and national levels to promote sound public policy and adequate funding for initiatives that prevent blindness and save sight. The annual "Eyes on Capitol Hill" event provides vision advocates an opportunity to meet with congressional leaders and policymakers.

SeniorNet

571-203-7100
www.seniornet.org

SeniorNet provides older adults with education and access to computer technologies to enhance their lives and enable them to share their knowledge and wisdom. The organization supports about 200 Learning Centers throughout the United States and in other countries. The website provides a list of these centers, organized by state and country. These centers offer introductory courses on computers, word processing, the Internet, and email. The centers are housed in a variety of locations such as senior centers, community centers, public libraries, schools and colleges, and clinics and hospitals. SeniorNet also offers easy-to-understand online lessons in using a computer, including utilizing accessibility options. In addition, the organization offers discounts on computer-related and other products and services.

SeniorNet publishes newsletters and a variety of other instructional materials, collaborates in research on older adults and technology, and holds regional conferences for volunteers.

Government agencies—programs, services, and eligibility

The Assistive Technology Act, enacted by Congress in 1998, is commonly known as the "Tech Act." Funding authorized by the Tech Act supports general types of programs, which vary from state to state: grant programs, protection and advocacy services, and alternative financing programs for purchasing assistive technology. The Tech Act provides services to those who live with virtually any type of disability for these people's full lifespans.

Some government agencies have special programs for people who are eligible for services if they meet the agencies' strict definition of "blind." If you meet one of the following criteria, you may qualify for these programs.

- Even with glasses or contact lenses, you cannot see better than 20/200 in your better eye.
- Your field of vision is 20 degrees or less.

Although people with macular disease may never reach this stage of vision loss, information on some of the major programs is included here nevertheless. It is possible that there could be some flexibility in applying the criteria.

Department of Veterans Affairs, VHA Optometry Service, Low Vision Rehabilitation

www.va.gov/BLINDREHAB/VIST.asp
202-461-7317

The VHA Optometry Service offers a wide variety of services along the continuum of visual impairment ranging from primary eye and low vision care to Visual Impairment Center to Optimize Remaining Sight (VICTORS) programs and Blind Rehabilitation Centers (BRCs). Optometrists help visually impaired veterans maintain functionality and independence by diagnosing levels of decreased vision and prescribing a variety of low vision devices such as specialized lens designs and prescriptions, pocket and hand held magnifiers, prismatic eyeglasses, telescopes, special lighting, and non-optical devices such as Closed Circuit Televisions (CCTVs) and head-mounted displays.

Internal Revenue Service

800-829-1040

www.irs.gov/publications/p554/ch04.htmld0e2715

If you meet IRS criteria for eligibility, you can receive an income tax deduction for blindness that is equal to the deduction for being over 65 years old. To claim the deduction for "partly blind," you must have a statement certified by your eye doctor or registered optometrist that declares one of the following:

- Even with glasses or contact lenses, you cannot see better than 20/200 in your better eye, or;

- Your field of vision is 20 degrees or less.

For many older and visually impaired taxpayers, the "over 65" and "blind" deductions result in more of a tax break than they would get if they itemized deductions, including expenses incurred as a result of vision impairment. And they definitely require a lot less work on the tax form than itemizing.

Medicare and Medicaid Services (Centers for)

800-633-4227

www.cms.hhs.gov

Services covered by Medicare depend on the specific plan you have and whether or not you are also covered by

Medicaid. Coverage varies from plan to plan, but services may include doctor visits, prescription drug coverage, coverage of costs incurred with eye injections, surgery for drooping eyelids or eyebrows, and mobility training. Check with your provider for information on the vision-related services that are covered in your plan.

National Eye Institute (NEI), Information Office, National Institutes of Health

301-496-5248
www.nei.nih.gov

The NEI was founded by Congress in 1968. It conducts research and education programs and provides information on eye diseases. See the web pages, Health Information, with an alphabetical list of eye diseases, and Education Programs. The National Eye Institute's Office of Communication, Health Education, and Public Liaison respond directly to requests for information on eye diseases and vision research.

National Council of State Agencies for the Blind (NCSAB)

www.ncsab.org/

Each state has a governmental agency to serve the needs of the blind and visually handicapped. The NCSAB is a national organization for these agencies and provides a forum for its members, including a directory of agencies listed by state. These agencies have various names, including State Services for the Blind and Visually Handicapped, Division of Rehabilitation Services; Blind Services, Department of Human Services; Aid to the Aged, Blind or Disabled; Board of Education and Services for the Blind; Board of Education and Services for the Blind. Each state provides services to the visually handicapped, but the governmental organizations themselves and the services they provide vary from state to state.

Services that may be provided include:

- Vocational rehabilitation and job placement services
- Financial assistance or referrals to other agencies and organizations that provide similar services in the community
- Orientation and mobility training and transportation
- Communication center that has a special library and transcription service, providing reading material in alternate formats to citizens who have difficulty reading normal print
- Provision of playback machines for the Talking Book Program

Manufacturers and Distributors of Assistive Technology Products

THE PRODUCTS described in Chapter 9 are generally available from at least one of the three low vision stores listed in Appendix B. This Appendix contains a list of representative manufacturers and U.S. distributors of these products as of 2011.

Assistive technology is developing at such a rapid pace, with a steady stream of new products coming to market, that any list of specific products available is likely to become outdated quickly. Use the contact information below to help you find the latest devices and software that are currently on the market from these companies. Note: Some manufacturers are listed more than once because they make products in more than one category. You can also consult the AFB's (American Foundation for the Blind) website at www.afb.org/ for up-to-date lists of products and manufacturers. Enter "Products" in the search box. The AFB website also features reviews of assistive products. Enter "Product evaluations" in the search box.

Scanner Readers, Desktop

Guerilla Technologies
www.guerillatechnologies.com

Scanner Readers, Portable

Enhanced Vision
www.enhancedvision.com

K-NFB Reading Technology, Inc.
www.knfbreader.com

Readers/Magnifiers, Portable Multifunction

Guerilla Technologies
www.guerillatechnologies.com

Software, Internet-Access (No Typing Required)

Serotek Corporation
www.serotek.com

Software, Magnification/Screen Reading (Typing Required)

Ai Squared
www.aisquared.com
This company produces ZoomText, integrated
   magnification and screen reading software.

Dolphin Computer Access, Ltd.
www.yourdolphin.com
This British company produces both screen
   magnification and screen reading software.

Freedom Scientific
www.freedomscientific.com
This company produces both screen magnification
   JAWS® screen reading software.

Software, Speech Transcription

Nuance
www.nuance.com
Speech Scribe is an advanced personal transcription
   solution for the Mac.

Text to Speech Software

Adobe Reader
www.adobe.com

Optelec
www.optelec.com

Desktop and Portable Video Magnifiers (CCTVs)

Freedom Vision
www.freedomvision.net

Human Ware
(Headquarters: Australia)
www.humanware.com

Optelec
www.optelec.com

Video Magnifiers, Handheld

Enhanced Vision
www.enhancedvision.com

Acknowledgments

WRITING THIS BOOK while living with gradually decreasing vision has not been a solo journey. I've received support and inspiration along the way from the many guides listed here.

I am deeply grateful to the staff at Vision Loss Resources in Minneapolis, including Ellen Morrow, MA, and her support group members; Kate Grathwol, PhD; Jean Christy; the class instructors, and my fellow skills class students.

My thanks to the many medical professionals who have provided both excellent care over the years and invaluable support and supplemental information for this book, including my ophthalmologist, Dorothy Horns, MD; my retinologist, Robert C. Ramsay, MD; and clinical research coordinator Julianne Enloe, CCRP, COA; my primary care physician, Louise G. Wright, MD; my audiologist, Julie A. Klosterman, MS, CCC-A; and my Pilates instructor, Angela Kneale, OTR, Certified Pilates Instructor.

My thanks to dear friends who have assisted in this project in multiple ways: Rosemary Kokesh, Arlys Gribovsky, Diane Follmer, Nancy Quinlan, Sharon Nelson, Reiko Ito Shellum-Koeck and Eugene Koeck, Amy Krane, "Taxi Al" Perlman, Jeanette DesMarais, and Mary Salisbury.

Thanks also to my talented publishing team, who helped bring this book to a high professional level: my editors, Linda Gray and Marly Cornell, designer Monica Baziuk, photographer Scott Knutson, indexer Robert J. Richardson, proofreader Maggie Gallivan, and Mary Rowles at Independent Publishers Group.

My heartfelt gratitude goes to my family for their support from the moment I had the idea of writing this book. Thanks to my son, Steven Wolfe, for his photography and for assuming management responsibilities in our publishing business to free my time for writing; to my daughter, Katie Wolfe, my planning buddy who kept me on track while having some fun along the way; and to my sister, Jean Richter, for reviewing endless drafts and providing emotional support when I was discouraged. To my late husband, Fancher E. Wolfe, my most poignant thanks for continuing to support my writing, even as his health declined.

About the author

PEGGY R. WOLFE is uniquely qualified to write a book about living with vision loss. Her expertise with macular disease dates back to the 1950s when her uncle became legally blind and she read aloud his favorite books. In the early 1980s, her mother discovered after cataract surgery that the underlying cause of her vision loss was macular degeneration. Peggy helped by writing checks, shopping, errands, companionship, and placing orders for her mother's beloved Talking Books. Then, in 1999, at the age of sixty-nine, Peggy was diagnosed with macular degeneration.

Writing a book about what she has learned, and continues to learn, was a natural choice. Peggy's father authored how-to books on electrical wiring and she serves as the president of the publishing company he founded. An English and philosophy major in college, she earned a master's degree in library science. She established the corporate library at The Pillsbury Company and later worked as a research fellow/librarian at the University of Minnesota. She volunteers in her church's music department, takes ballet class through her school district's adult enrichment program, and studies Pilates and kettlebells with private instructors. She gives presentations on her book at senior centers and teaches short courses in community education programs. When Peggy celebrated her eightieth birthday in 2010, she developed a new slogan, "Eighty Power!"

She lives in Minnetonka, Minnesota.

Index

Transportation services,
continued

Taxi Al (My Story),
176–177

Typing

keyboards, computer,
155–156

software, 159–160

typing skills, refreshing,
154

■ V

Veterans Affairs, Blind
Rehabilitation
Service, 210–211

Video magnifiers (CCTVs)

desktop, 151

handheld, 150–151,
152

suppliers of, 215–218

Vision Loss Resources,
Minneapolis, 146

Vision testing

Amsler grid, 13

doctor visits, 15–17

fluorescein angiography,
16

OCT (ocular coherence
tomography), 16

research study (My
Story), 20–21

self-testing, 13–14

Visual field, 22, 24

Vitamins, 19–20

Volunteering, My Story,
11–12

■ W

Wills

procrastination and
my husband's will,
137–140

writing a will, 129–130

See also Attorneys

1496

Order Book

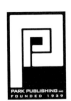

Phone 1-800-841-0383
Fax 715-246-4366
Email parkpublishing@nrmsinc.com
Park Publishing, Inc.
511 Wisconsin Drive
New Richmond, WI 54017–2613

COPIES	DISCOUNT	PRICE PER COPY
Single	—	$17.95 + $3.50 shipping
2–5	20%	$14.36 + shipping
6–10	30%	$12.56 + shipping
11–50	40%	$10.77 + shipping

For over 50 copies, call 1-800-841-0383 for discounts

Please send the following, based on above discounts.

#_____ copies @ $_____ = $ _____

Shipping by UPS Ground will be added for two or more copies
Sales tax: Minnesota residents add 6.875% sales tax

Name _____

Address _____

City _____ State _____ ZIP _____

Phone _____ Email _____

Send check, money order, or credit card information
VISA, MasterCard, American Express, or Discover card

Name on card _____

Card number _____ Exp _____ / _____

Security verification _____ (last 3 digits back of card)